THE
MOTHER
MANTRA

THE MOTHER MANTRA

The Ancient Shamanic Yoga of Non-Duality

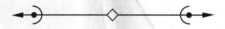

Selene Calloni Williams

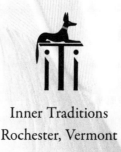

Inner Traditions
Rochester, Vermont

Inner Traditions
One Park Street
Rochester, Vermont 05767
www.InnerTraditions.com

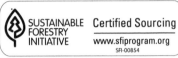

Text stock is SFI certified

Originally published in Italian under the title *Mantra madre, la tradizione e le
pratiche segrete del matrimonio mistico e del risveglio* by Edizioni Mediterranee,
Via Flaminia, 109-00196, Roma

First English edition published in 2015 under the title *Mother Mantra: Tradition
and Secret Practices of the Mystical Marriage and of Reawakening* by Edizioni
Mediterranee

First U.S. edition published in 2019 by Inner Traditions

Cataloging-in-Publication Data is available from the Library of Congress

ISBN 978-1-62055-792-1 (print)
ISBN 978-1-62055-793-8 (ebook)

Printed and bound in the United States by Lake Book Manufacturing, Inc.
The text stock is SFI certified. The Sustainable Forestry Initiative® program
promotes sustainable forest management.

10   9   8   7   6   5   4   3   2   1

Text design and layout by Virginia Scott Bowman
This book was typeset in Garamond Premier Pro and Futura with Centaur and
Avenir used as display typefaces
Translation by Selene Calloni Williams
Illustrations by Gabriele Albanese

To send correspondence to the author of this book, mail a first-class letter to the
author c/o Inner Traditions • Bear & Company, One Park Street, Rochester, VT
05767, and we will forward the communication, or contact the author directly at
selenecalloniwilliams.com/english-version.

Contents

The Key to the Reabsorption of Reality

FOR ANY ESOTERIC PATH, journey of self-development or personal growth, alchemy, or depth psychology to be truly effective, it must harbor in its core the extraordinary key of the "reabsorption of reality." Shamanism, yoga, tantric Buddhism, Christian Gnosticism, the Kabbalah, Sufism, and the esoteric religions are all founded on the same key, the same procedure.

To "reabsorb reality" means to make room for the soul. Indeed, it means taking every thing, person, object, or place that we come into contact with daily and bringing it back to its true nature, which is image. Even physics shows us that everything is image, dream, apparition. Matter, in the sense of substance, is an illusion. The electron is a wave that propagates in emptiness, even though to our senses it is a particle. We humans are so fearful of the void, by which we mean the natural principle, that we are unable to perceive it, but we may conceive it between our heart and mind. Matter is not substance but soul; that is, pure emptiness.

This process of reabsorption, also defined as the "withdrawal of projections," is the path that enables us to unburden ourselves of the weight of objective matter, of unavoidable events to which we must succumb. The path of reabsorption of reality leads us to become masters, partners, lovers of the events—which are beings, entities, spirits—and it awakens us from the illusion of being in the role of victims. The path of reabsorption of reality is the path of the aesthetic experience as the main alternative to the unaesthetic experience, caused by therapy.

For this reason the process of withdrawing projections is considered "the means." It is indeed the means to a free and fulfilled life. It is, actually, a very simple and natural means, so simple indeed that the difficulty in achieving and using it lies only in our ability to deconstruct our self, in order to tap in to it. However society and its institutions, being themselves structures, are always in opposition to deconstruction. Thus, from ancient times this "means" has always traveled nonconventional routes, far from the central institutions.

This "means" is best expressed in its purest and most original form, with no superstructure, by the Mother Mantra tradition. It has traveled the routes of tantric-shamanic yoga and alchemy for many centuries now, both in the East and West. The name Mother Mantra is a choice. In the past it has been defined as the "psychic formula of the imaginal creation";* others have referred to it as the "magic formula"; others have defined it as "the automatic means," or simply "the means."

The roots of the tradition of the Mother Mantra, like those of alchemy and tantrism, are lost in time. Even though the classification of these traditions was written in historically datable times, it cannot be denied that this codification was based on oral traditions that had been passed down from ancient times. Polytheist and animist populations who lived in symbiosis with nature and its deities passed on their knowledge, perceptions, and rituals of nature through the great esoteric paths. This is probably why some scholars have sought connections between tantrism, alchemy, and animistic shamanism.

---

*In this context *imaginal* relates to the liminal threshold between the conscious and the subconscious, where images are produced. In depth psychology the imaginal tradition refers to the complexity of images, myths, and rites on which a culture is founded.

Even though there is no proof of a common historical root, there is such a deep-felt continuity between shamanism, tantrism, and alchemy as to strongly point to one big common tradition that takes on different hues—some extremely intuitive, some rather refined and learned. We may say that tantrism and alchemy are the learned forms by which shamanic, tribal, ancestral traits have been expressed through history, both in the East and West. Tantrism and alchemy transmit the message of our origins, enriching it with cults, practices, traditions, rituals, myths, and wisdom.

Depth psychology, which is connected to polytheist and shamanic visions (such as in James Hillman's archetypal or polytheist psychology), is also a conscious transmission tool of the "means." There is a golden thread that ties the revealed knowledge of the origins to the esoteric and spiritual traditions, weaving up to depth psychology.

The Mother Mantra tradition is this priceless golden thread. This is the precious treasure that I share in the following pages, with the permission of the visible and invisible masters. The Mother Mantra has the power of being universal, yet at the same time adapts perfectly well to the culture of the practitioner. Universality implies that it is for any- and everyone, regardless of religion, ethnicity, or culture. Particularity refers to its ability to adapt and fit perfectly to the folds of the single practitioner's psyche.

The Mother Mantra presents three forms, called "variants": two universal variants and a particular one. The three variants are basically three mantras for reabsorption. The first of these three mantras is the properly said Mother Mantra. The second is the Egyptian Mantra. The third is the Mystical Marriage Mantra.

The Egyptian Mantra and the Mystical Marriage Mantra are the two universal variants of the Mother Mantra and are presented in the pages that follow. The Egyptian Mantra allows harmony with the planet, with the Earth's rhythm and nature's abundance; furthermore, it tunes the conscious will to the shadow's will, a necessary step for the successful outcome of any of life's projects. The Mystical Marriage Mantra develops an intimate, erotic-creative union with the underworld bride/bridegroom, which confers inspiration and pleasure.

The Mother Mantra itself, the particular variant, is spread by the Mother Mantra Masters only and passed on solely to Guardians. A Guardian is someone who is not only interested in the personal practice of the Mother Mantra but also wishes to spread this mantra and its associated rituals. If the Mother Mantra is not received from a Guardian it will not produce the same effects. For that reason it is not revealed here.

A Carrier of the Mother Mantra is someone who has received initiation from a Guardian. When you seriously practice the spiritual exercises shared in this book you too will become a Carrier. The first two variants of the Mother Mantra may be practiced with full benefit by Carriers.

All three mantras of the Mother Mantra tradition enable us to retract our projections and to take responsibility for all the emotions and events that we have experienced in life. We may thus let go of our roles as victims of events and our reactions to them to become teachers, partners, and lovers of the events that are the multiple aspects of the invisible lover, which is our soul.

The mantras taught here allow reality to be reabsorbed. This enables the physical senses—which are managed by the mind and its value sets—to experience the substantial illusion of the world and the fundamental imaginal nature of every thing. Awareness is thus allowed to rise above the categories of good and bad, true and false, and flow freely in the infinite universe of beauty, in the state of nature.

The Mother Mantra has the power of a thousand hurricanes and a thousand storms unleashed together in the inner sky of our inseparable union with Everything. After this big bang, true life begins. The true birth is the second; the true mother is the second; the true life is the second.

In the first chapter, "Natural Spiritual Experience," natural tradition is contrasted with social tradition. The differences in worldview and life experience that result from the immersion in and adherence to one or the other are explored in detail, resulting in greater clarity about beauty and the good, death and immortality, power and fighting, and sacred and healing rituals.

This provides the necessary background to understand the experiences of the Great Image—the erotic creative union of the mystical marriage—presented in the second chapter, "The Great Image," dramatized by the author's explorations in widely different cultural settings around the world.

The third chapter, "The Underworld or Celestial Bride/ Bridegroom," invites us to the intimate understanding that both counterparts of the mystical marriage are within each of us and the energy and joy that are fostered by that understanding.

"The Four Movements of the Mother Mantra Tradition" presented in the fourth chapter are the core practices that have the power to reabsorb reality and reunite the divine lovers, leading to the awakening of the initiated. These include a number of significant psychic formulas, especially the two universal variants of the Mother Mantra: the Egyptian Mantra and the Mystical Marriage Mantra.

The Mother Mantra tradition also includes the application of the mantras in spiritual healing rituals and in several very effective spiritual exercises that open the body, mind, and heart to the revelation and an inspired life; these occur throughout the book and are highlighted in chapter 5, "The Spiritual Practices of the Morning and Evening," and chapter 8, "Further Spiritual Practices for Well-Being," which includes the creation of a visionary mandala and a ritual of self-healing.

In chapter 6, "Rite, Myth, and Compassion," you will meet the seven great messengers and learn how to understand their messages, to heed the soul's calling. This chapter also shares a crucial difference between therapy and the aesthetic experience of sacred ritual.

Chapter 7, "Freeing the Hostage Prometheus," explores the deep meaning of the ancient myth of "the enchained hero," representative of true knowledge and the love that leads to liberation. This chapter also includes practices of the Mother Mantra tradition that bring about spiritual revolution.

This book thus will endow you with the many blessings of the Mother Mantra tradition and will create a bridge to a new perception of reality.

1

Natural Spiritual Experience

THE RELIGION OF NATURE DIFFERS from social religions inasmuch as it doesn't bother to distinguish good from evil. It is animated by the observation and imitation of nature. If we observe nature we feel that the inspiring principle that moves it identifies more easily with beauty than with goodness, as commonly understood by humankind.

The parameters of good and bad, of true and false, right and wrong, and of all the other opposing pairs in the human mind, are not principles of the state of nature.

Nature moves toward beauty. Primitive religions, defined as religions of nature, express the harmony of beauty, not its goodness.

In Homer's times all the souls, whether good or bad, were together in the underworld. Then the Elysium appeared, and the fate of the good was separated from that of the so-called bad. According to the shamanic vision, the world is tripartite, with an underworld, a middle world, and a world of the skies. The world of the skies is the world of the deities and ideas, the middle world is the human world, and the underworld is the world of the dead, with no distinction between good and bad.

In Inca mythology we find a similar vision. The Incas believed in a world of three levels: Hanan Pacha, the "higher world," where the divinities reside; Kay Pacha or the "world that is," where the living beings reside; and Uku Pacha, or "the world below," where the souls of the dead and the unborn reside. Here again there is no distinction between good and bad.

The core experience of the religion of nature is the ecstasy that is born through immersion in nature itself. The secrets of natural religions are centered on techniques that bring about ecstatic experiences, such as in the shamanic trance, the trance of the tantric oracles, or the trance of the Pythia of Delphi. Pythia was a powerful prophetess who spoke for God, the spokeswoman of Apollo, and the high priestess of the Apollo temple at Delphi (in ancient Greece). Her prophecies were inspired or fueled by the spirit of God or by "Enthusiasmos." The trance puts the human in contact with nature's harmonies and laws, which are expressed in the revelation of beauty.

While the natural spiritual experience is always an ecstatic experience of beauty, this is overruled by the experience of good in the field of social religions.

Considering that we don't want to renounce good, yet we don't want to be robbed of beauty, let's ask ourselves on the one hand what beauty is and on the other what good is.

BEAUTY

Beauty is the soul of nature. Everything in nature moves toward beauty. What could be more beautiful than giving oneself?

In nature everything gives itself. According to Heraclitus, a person cannot bathe in the same river twice, because the second time the river has already given itself and no longer exists; another river has taken its place.

In nature everything gives itself; everything is evanescent, a shadow, a mirage that appears and immediately disappears. Impermanence is the main trait of nature. Why should nature give itself, if not for love? Beauty is the natural state, which is impermanence, love, giving.

Nature has its laws, which do not discriminate between the opposites (good, evil, right, wrong, true, false . . .). They are laws of harmony, of rhythm.

Giving oneself is the purest expression of beauty. Beauty is a state of sameness, complexity and instantaneity. These are important visions for those initiated into the Mother Mantra tradition.

Sameness

Sameness is a natural condition. Beauty, being balance, is sameness. Indeed, by the expression *sameness* we mean the perfect alignment of the opposites or, if you prefer, the contemporaneity of the opposites, or the state of being beyond good and evil.

Sameness is the perfect balance between the opposites: between father and mother, or female and male, which are symbols that sum up all the opposites.

Male is *logos* (word), order, logic, reason, radiance, evidence, the manifest, life, effort, conquest, penetration, foundation, support, salty, movement. Using Nietzsche's term, male is Apollonian.

Female is irrational, chaos, change, shadow, the non-manifest, death, inspiration, passivity, opening, fruit, sweet, stillness. To use another term from Nietzsche, female is Dionysian.

Instantaneity

Going back to the Heraclitus saying that a person cannot bathe twice in the same river, we may say that the river doesn't exist as a material object and that there are an infinite number of rivers, infinite images of the river. All the visible and invisible images of the river, its apparitions and shadows, are beyond time; they are in the simultaneity of the here and now and are always present, even though the human mind cannot grasp all of them because fear won't allow it to look into the shadow.

In the natural state everything is instantaneous: present here and now. The feeling that everything has its own story and continuity is an illusion created by the sense of "I," which is, in turn, illusion.

Complexity

Complexity is the same as instantaneity; it's another way of defining it. It means that each single appearance and disappearance of the river, its manifestations and shadows, are all one within the other, just like the images of a fractal or hologram. A fractal is a complex geometric pattern in which the pattern of the whole keeps recurring, in smaller and smaller fragments seen through a magnifying glass.

To better explain the complexity of reality, as an example I often share an episode a friend told me, which illustrates the deception that the mind undergoes.

One day my friend told me that she had been to Hong Kong for a session of regressive hypnosis during which she had seen herself dying during childbirth on a blood-stained bed. "Now I understand why I don't want to have children in this life," she said. "And I understand why I kept on having the same nightmare as a child: I would dream that I was running happily in a meadow until the anxious crying of a baby would wake me up in terror. It's probably why I'm named after my paternal grandmother, who died during her third childbirth."

The idea of a linear path of time and the cause-and-effect logic are social myths that effect the perception of reality creating a deception of the mind. My friend established a logical and temporal sequence of cause and effect for a series of images that are actually eternally simultaneous. In the depth of my friend's psyche there is an archetype; that is, an original image, an original impression from which all the others are produced: that of the dying woman, the dying grandmother, and so on. All of the images are in the instantaneity of sameness, in the here and now, reflected in a unique image, the totality and power of which can't be grasped by the "I," which needs to filter the vision gradually, thus creating the impression of a before and an after, causing the deception of the mind.

Complexity means that the all is in the part and the part is in the all. Interactivity and adaptability are further traits of complex systems.

Interactivity refers to the fact that all parts of nature interact with one another. They interact and modify each other.

Adaptability is a natural principle that is quite well known. If a significant part of the system changes then the rest changes to adapt to the system's change.

Critical Mass

Another important concept that arises from the observation of the natural state is that of the *critical mass*. To change a complex system a significant part of it needs to be modified. Complex interactive systems—take a family, for example—are such that if a significant part of the system changes, so does the whole system. How much poison must be poured into a river to say that the whole river is poisoned? According to the homeopathic principle a drop would be enough; the intention alone would suffice.

So we should reformulate the question in the following way: How much poison is it necessary to pour into the river to bring about a mutation that can be perceived by the human senses? This amount of poison is what we define as the *critical mass*. The critical mass is the amount or intensity of a mutation that must come about in a part of a system so as to produce a transformation of the system as a whole that can be perceived by the human senses.

GOOD

Good is a concept produced by the human mind. It cannot be found anywhere in nature, if not in the human mind. Good is based on permanence: good means staying, not dying, not vanishing. Dying, vanishing, ending is "bad." Living, remaining visible, is good for the individual.

While we wait to see what death actually is, it is perceived as something evil by the living. Because of this fear of death, of shadow, of invisibility, the human mind creates an impression of the material object, which is what lasts, which has continuity.

The body, which is a symbol, an image, or a vehicle of pure apparition as defined in Buddhism, ends up being perceived as a material object. And the same goes for the river in which the body bathes, or for any other aspect of nature.

So if we have to say what good is, we must say that it is what the impression of materialism and the objectivity of things is based upon. This impression is very dear to the human mind; that is, it generates attachment because it enables a person to produce yet another impression: that of having power over body and nature.

A material object that has continuity can be analyzed, calculated, predicted, measured. The human mind may exercise power over material nature. But material nature doesn't exist; it is an illusion born from the mind itself out of fear, anxiety, out of the fear of giving itself, of vanishing, of loving, out of its need for control.

DEATH

If beauty is giving oneself, and if giving oneself is impermanence, and impermanence is love, then death, which is the most intense and intrinsic impermanence, is love.

Death is love. Love is that which awakens from the big illusion of materialism, donating freedom, bliss, and immortality.

Death is the passage to immortality.

We have seen how the materialistic vision is shaped from discrimination, from the separation of the opposites, good, bad, right, wrong, true, false, life, death. A material object cannot be both alive and dead at the same time.

Individuals, hypnotized by their own minds, cannot be living and dying simultaneously, just as they cannot see the world both on this side and that side of the Great Threshold: they can either see this side or that side.

As a human being gradually manages to come free from the hypnosis of materialism one becomes able to perceive one's own body as a symbol and not as an object. The symbol exists simultaneously on both sides of the Great Threshold, as it is pure energy, willpower, desire, aspiration, love. It is not an object.

The awakened human being partakes in a condition of natural love wherein death, as perceived by those still under hypnosis, doesn't exist. The dying and the living may possibly exist, the former passing through the realms of the shadows beyond the Great Threshold and the latter passing through the realms of the visible this side of the Great Threshold. The dying and the living appear simultaneously to the eyes of the awakened.

This process of unveiling is progressive, with growing levels of intensity. The more intense it is, the more the person undergoing it feels free from fear. The more fear is overcome, the weaker becomes the need to control and manage reality, and consequently the weaker becomes the need to measure reality by its opposites (good, bad, life, death, and so on), and one can plunge into beauty, which is love.

THE SACRED AND RITUAL

Giving oneself, which is the purest expression of beauty, is the *sacrum facere* (making sacred). Sacred is to give oneself, and to give oneself is sacred. This is perfectly illustrated in several populations' rituals of sacrifice. Ritual sacrifice is the moment when a human being totally partakes of the natural state. It is the moment in which the human being understands and celebrates nature and its will to give itself and to love.

The sacred exists in beauty, which is the state of sameness and instantaneity. When the sacred is not in sameness it is deviant. Sameness is the perfect balance between the opposites, between Mother and Father.

In cultures dominated by a matriarch-centered symbolism—for example Maya, Inca, Hindu—the sacred has been over-weighted toward the feminine, so the ritual sacrifices implied human sacrifice. This is a female deviation from the sacred.

In cultures—such as ours—dominated by a patriarch-centered symbolism, the sacred is dominated by the need for control, analysis, management. The loss of the sacred is the loss of communion with nature. Individuals in our culture are eco-incompatible. For them nature is a resource to be exploited. And even when they try to be environmentally oriented, their effort is focused on organizing the exploitation of the planet methodically so as to be able to keep on exploiting it. Ecology, in a patriarch-centered paradigm of reality, is always anthropocentric; it is centered on the survival of humans and their needs.

In a culture centered on the instantaneity of sameness—classic Greek culture might fit as example—the sacrificial ritual is expressed through art. Real art—which doesn't exist in desacralized cultures—is the highest form of sacrifice, inasmuch as it manifests the full understanding and partaking of the natural state. Real art is the expression of the human being in full harmony with nature.

In a culture centered on the instantaneity of sameness, art is prayer, healing, and enlightenment; it has a cathartic, thaumaturgic, and ecstatic effect. Through art—think of Greek sculpture—deities are depicted and honored. Through art—think of Greek theater—psychotherapy is done. Through art—think of the myths and Greek poetry—the ecstatic experience is born, which is the experience of full immersion in universal love, by which beauty is expressed.

POWER

Human beings stop doing the sacrificial rites and leave the sacred because they want power. They want control over nature and their own body. Knowledge can give them this power. Knowledge bent on power exists in a distinct manner, separate from love. This knowledge is a technical knowledge functional to power. It is a desacralized knowledge, which creates an unnatural world of conflict and obscurity. Knowledge coupled with love is the knowledge of the sacred, of giving oneself and of beauty; thus it is a knowledge dedicated to the search for truth rather than to power.

The myth of the man bent on power who chooses a discriminatory knowledge is often found throughout religious literature. Think of the apple of Adam and Eve or the lay myth of Minos. Minos, the mythical king of Crete, represents that part of our psyche that desires power and control over body and nature. Minos asks Poseidon, who represents the divinity of nature, for a sign of the fact that he may have power. Poseidon concedes him this sign in the form of a white bull, with the agreement that Minos will give the bull back through a ritual sacrifice. But when Minos sees the power and beauty of the bull, he decides to keep it for himself and introduces it into his herd.

This attempt at taming the wild is a cultural archetype that we all harbor in the depth of our psyche. But above all, what we carry within us is the ancestral betrayal of our pact with nature, which ruptured the universal balance.

We well know the consequences of this gesture because we are forced to live separate from the original purity of every single thing; we belong to a culture with a sense of sin, of guilt, founded on a hyperbolic separation of good and evil and on the desperate run from an unexplainable obscurity that we feel is following us.

We are running from the gods who are our own psychic depths, who are the images that mold us, of which we are made; they are our organs and our soul. The gods are eidola, ideas. They are the lords of nature, all one in another, all part of a complex universe. All the gods are the irate Poseidon responding to the betrayal of Minos. In the myth, angry Poseidon makes Pasiphae, Minos's wife, fall in love with the white bull. Pasiphae makes Daedalus construct a wooden mare, into which she shuts herself to couple with the white bull. The Minotaur is born from them, a monstrous beast, half man and half bull.

The desire to maintain control is a cultural habit perpetuated by technical knowledge, which is bent on power. Indeed, Minos then forces Daedalus to build the labyrinth in which the Minotaur is trapped. But the Minotaur asks for the yearly sacrifice of seven young boys and girls for him to devour. So the sacrifice, left unaccomplished by a broken promise, becomes deviant. This mirrors the state of our society, which finds it hard to live with the shadows that disturb it and falls ill.

Thus the gods become social and individual evils. The gods become illnesses, starting with the great Pan, who becomes panic, anxiety, depression.

Theseus, the Greek hero who travels from Athens to Crete to slaughter the Minotaur, is once again the "I," which in the human psyche represents the structure that yearns for power. Theseus kills the Minotaur with the help of Ariadne, who gives him the well-known red ball of thread to find his way out of the labyrinth. Ariadne represents the maiden who falls in love with the wrong man after separation from her own instinct, symbolized by her brother, the Minotaur. Theseus wants to take her with him, but during the return journey to Athens, when his ship is moored off the island of Naxos for the night, he abandons the sleeping Ariadne. The young woman, who, on waking, has to face being abandoned and in mortal danger, represents the soul or instinct, which, to find itself again, must descend to the underworld and face the night of solitude.

Poseidon, irate, unleashes a wind strong enough to rip and tear the sails of Theseus's ship, so he has to hoist the black sails he carried instead. When his father, King Aegeus, sees the black sails as the ship comes closer, he is convinced that they are a sign of the death of Theseus and throws himself into the sea, which now takes his name. Theseus becomes king of Athens. He has the power of the ruler—his name shares its root with the Greek word *thesmos,* meaning "institution"—but his private life is disastrous: his wife hangs herself, and his son Hippolytus dies because of a curse of Theseus himself. After adventures, feats, and travels—including the descent to Hades where he fails to kidnap Persephone—he comes to an unworthy end for a hero. Indeed, when he returns to Athens he discovers that he has been dethroned by Menestheus. Theseus tries to drive out the usurper in vain and so takes refuge on the island of Skyros, the land of King Lycomedes. Jealous of the fame of his illustrious guest, Lycomedes schemes to get rid of him. With the excuse of showing him the extent of his domains, he leads Theseus to a steep cliff and throws him over the edge.

According to Virgil, after his death Theseus undergoes the same punishment he had received when in life he made the descent to Hades to try to kidnap Persephone, only this time for eternity.

THE SURVIVAL INSTINCT

The survival instinct is the fundamental component of the sacred. It is not to be confused with the fear of death. The fear of death arises out of a lack of love. Love leads you to talk to the rain, the rivers and the trees, the cliffs and the birds; it leads you onto a common path, to a universal communion able, in turn, to conceive the will to vanish into everything, to give oneself, and to enjoy the impermanence without which it would be impossible to give oneself in every instant. The survival instinct is the assertion of impermanence, inasmuch as everything in this world is asserted thanks to its opposite, and a force to be exerted needs a resistance.

The fear of death is tied to the deceptive idea of oneself as an individual separate from the whole. The survival instinct is the assertion of the sacred; it is that which allows the exercise of the ability to give oneself. That there may be less awareness in a deer's or in a tiger's giving itself than in a human's giving himself or herself is a human judgment.

The awareness of giving oneself is not necessarily related to the attachment to the idea of "I am."

The Carrier of the Mother Mantra

A person initiated in the knowledge of the Mother Mantra tradition is a Carrier of the Mantra. Such a person has a strong survival instinct; indeed, one of the "promises" made by the initiate is to live a long life in good health (in chapter 5 we will explain the promises). The initiates' survival instinct is proportional to the ability to give oneself, and both increase over the time one does the practices of the Mother Mantra tradition. At the same time one's fear of death diminishes as the illusion of being separate from the All dissolves. Freedom in life is undoubtedly a life lived without fear. The unconscious fear of death influences every aspect of human behavior; the relationship with others and ourselves is founded on it.

The fear of death is a main player in our relationships with our partners and with money; it strongly conditions our state of psycho-physical health, daily stress, quality of rest, eating habits, and minor and major choices in life. The subconscious fear of death governs our relationship with the gods, with ideas. When it is very strong we live on a purely analytical and mental plane where ideas are sterile, whereas in the absence of fear ideas are full of love and fertile.

Depth psychology shows that the fear of death underlies every human problem, because death is the ultimate secret of our nature, and also our beginning: we come from a universe of invisibility, and the kingdom of Hades is where we are headed.

The Particular Variant of the Mother Mantra

The particular variant of the Mother Mantra has the sole purpose of meeting and reabsorbing the images—that is, the archetypes—peculiar to each culture. Thus there is a Western variant tied to the Jewish Christian tradition, a variant tied to the Muslim tradition, a variant tied to the Buddhist tradition, and one tied to the Hindu tradition. There are also variants for ethnic, cultural, and religious minority groups.

Indeed, over the centuries, the differing traditions have undoubtedly created differing imaginal traditions to which the populations have unconsciously adapted. Individuals are governable, measurable, and predictable as long as the symbols of their own cultural background act within them automatically, even filtering their perceptions and forcing them to see, hear, touch, smell, and taste according to a given set of values that align the senses—mental operations—with the standard functions and answers common to that culture. From a dialectic point of view, freedom is freedom from something, so our possibility of freedom is tied to the existence of a world that is not free.

In any given social tradition founded on categories of power, it is possible to access a powerful and infallible Mother Mantra, capable of reabsorbing the fundamental images—that is, the archetypes on which the traditions are built—capable of guiding the human beings of that society to freedom. However the particular variant is passed on solely from master to disciple by word of mouth through a traditional and personal initiation process.

If the Mother Mantra is received from a Guardian, an initiation is accomplished, which implies the transmission of an energy and the opening of a path. Since ancient times an initiation has been an investiture that allows obstacles, created by the social and mental structures, to be more easily overcome. Thanks to this received initiation the practice of the two universal variants of the Mother Mantra will implement a progressive and certain awakening. These simple but fundamental principles ensure that the Mother Mantra is spread safely.

The knowledge of the apex of the Mother Mantra is kept secret to protect it, because those uninterested in freedom could harm it, and it would possibly take centuries to mend. How can knowledge become damaged? By mocking it—as has been tried over the centuries with the tantric teachings—by debasing, distorting, and discrediting it.

Having or not having the knowledge of the third variant of the Mother Mantra and the initiation to the role of Guardian doesn't influence the efficacy of the practice in itself, but the knowledge does influence the efficacy of the spreading of the practice. Indeed, the knowledge of the particular variant of the Mother Mantra activates further knowledge, which enables the Guardians to transmit the two universal variants in complete safety.

THE CALCULATION OF PERSONAL ADVANTAGE AND DISADVANTAGE

The parameters of good and evil, health and illness, and so on, on which the mind focuses, are socially induced. Nature moves toward beauty, not goodness, which is a concept created by the human mind. To achieve power the mind creates its own scale of values with the aim of making nature and the body controllable, measurable, predictable, and governable.

The knowledge used to achieve power and control—not love and self-giving—is exerted through theories that express a technical kind of know-how, which is aimed at power. This technical know-how is the knowledge of a mental model of reality, not of natural reality, which is pure emptiness, impermanence, self-giving, beauty, love. It is not correct to state that natural reality is unknowable; it is knowable through love, through becoming that which is known.

The problem with technical knowledge aimed at control is that the supporting theories can be manipulated. Because the concepts of good, health, and truth are abstract they can thus be manipulated. When one makes an effort to think about one's own well-being or health, one doesn't *actually* think about one's own well-being or health at all but rather about the well-being and health of the system that determines the models of health and well-being.

So the world can essentially be grouped into two categories of people: those who believe in social values and respect them, and those who have understood that such values have no reason to exist in nature. In the latter category we find magicians, artists, hermits, ascetics, monks, and spiritual persons.

Deviation

The freedom from the hypnotism generated by the values of good and evil might be thought to imply a great risk, that of slipping adrift toward deviation, which is a lack of control such as in madness, greed, perversion, Satanism.

All these traits are the consequence of the exacerbated control and pressure of the values of good and evil, not of freedom. The natural energies are suppressed by the exertion of mental control out of fear and the lack of love and beauty. When the psyche's natural forces are overcompressed, a sort of psychosis arises, with thought drifting inexorably toward the thirst for power, perversion, and other deviant manifestations.

In our society the possibility of achieving power goes hand in hand with a psyche affected by lucid madness. When the gods, which are our most powerful psychic forces, our ideas, are not recognized but repressed, they end up over-running the mind and taking hold of reality in a devastating manner.

Balance in the Psyche and the World

The gods transcend the sphere of individuality. We must think of the gods in depersonalized terms. If the gods blow the minds of certain individuals, leading them to commit heinous crimes in the name of crazy religious, economic, or political theories, it is without doubt because there are other individuals in another part of the world who are strongly repressing natural energies, failing to recognize the wild dimension of the psyche in an attempt to dominate nature and the world.

Balance in the psyche and in the world is to be considered with a mind free from the sense of individuality and materialism. Just as a person can be overcome by the forces of his own psyche, which he tries to repress out of fear, so is the world overridden by the very energies it wants to control.

THE TWO WAYS OF FIGHTING

The gods are always fighting each other, but the fight of the gods is not the fight of the individuals. Life in nature is a fight, but the fight in nature is not an artificial conflict of the mind.

In nature the guilt complex doesn't exist; the fight is for expressing beauty. Beauty is a touching universal experience; it is pathos, it is soul. We say that a plant, a mountain, or a tiger has a soul when it seems able to feel emotion. The soul is beauty and beauty is emotion.

Self-giving is the ultimate emotion, which is the purest expression of love. The natural fight for survival is the manifestation of beauty, devoid of guilt or prejudice. Individuals fight under manipulation, triggered by the theories of good and bad, right and wrong, true and false.

A wise person, a spiritual person, is not one who no longer fights but one who fights for love. Such a one doesn't suffer the conflict, is not weakened by the blows of the enemy, is not angry with the enemy, is not feeling judgment or guilt. Such a person doesn't fight for a system but for the soul.

The true spiritualist, just like Arjuna in the Bhagavad Gita, does not give up the fight. He knows that everything is perfect just as it is, that actually there is nothing to change in the world. He expresses himself in battle to manifest beauty, just as an artist expresses himself or herself in a work of art. The battle of the spiritualist, like that of the artist, does not give rise to suffering but instead to continual regeneration.

The free person fights for the emotion of love; the battle is creative, not destructive. The individual fights laboriously for personal advantage, without realizing that the mind that is calculating the personal pros and cons is, in actual fact, a tool that is and can be manipulated. Consequently such individuals fight for the system, even when they believe they are fighting against it.

Health and Sickness

When a free person falls ill he or she wonders what kind of emotion the illness will bring with it. Such persons delve into their own illness to search for the repressed sentiment: they look for it, love it, free it, live it, and sublimate it into the ecstasy of love between the human being and the Divine. Free individuals recognize the illness as the call of the shadows. And they bravely walk toward those shadows.

The shadows beckon when a primeval balance, a universal order, has been broken and needs to be reestablished. Beauty is harmony between light and shadow, death and life, dreaming and awaking.

When this harmony is shattered because, for example, one has forgotten one's invisible soul and has over-pursued the material values of the world, then the soul beckons from the world of invisibility, and its voice appears in the visible world in the form of disease, unease, and difficulty.

The spiritual person recognizes this and celebrates the call of the soul by venturing into the shadows, giving oneself up to the emotions that come with this, going the distance with the troubling experience that self-giving is, that beauty is.

Social individuals only want to sedate the call of the soul and anesthetize the voice of the gods, which are expressed through their own organs. The imperative function of any therapy is to soothe the soul's impact on life, keeping control—that is, the illusion of power—over body and nature.

The social individual generally chooses the therapeutic path. The free person generally chooses the aesthetic path. Both individuals may experience the same events; for example, both may choose surgery or medicine. What differs is the way each one lives the event. Pushed by fear, the social individual fights the illness to maintain control over one's own body, mind, life, and nature. Facing the same illness, the spiritual person fights to reestablish the balance between visible and invisible, to give back power to the soul.

The Ritual of Healing

Every time the primeval balance or universal order is broken; every time the deal with nature—the deal between Poseidon and Minos—is betrayed, every time beauty fails, then an illness, an unease, a disturbance, or a problem crops up, which has the task of putting things right.

In this sense our sicknesses, our disturbances, our unease, and our problems are indeed our biggest heritage: they are the voice of our soul calling from the realms of invisibility, the world beyond this world.

Once the balance has been broken on both sides the problem arises of where to direct our conscious attention: toward Minos, the "I" that wants control and power, or toward Poseidon, nature.

In truth, this problem can only be solved by reestablishing the balance between the "I" and nature and by developing an awareness that is well centered between the opposites. In duality one is overwhelmed. Duality implies either residing only in the mind or residing solely in the natural experience.

Take, for example, a person diagnosed with cancer who decides to entrust the management of his health solely to the so-called medical science. He will have made a unilateral choice of delegating the care of his health to a principle outside himself—doctors, drugs, surgery—a therapeutic principle based on a mental model of reality in which the body is a material object.

But a similar unilateral and unbalanced choice will also be made if a person decides to let nature run its course without having accomplished a true and proper healing ritual, confiding solely in the possibility that the body heals itself.

The path of sameness always implies a ritual for the reestablishment of the lost balance. This ritual must be perceived by every aspect of the person: body, feelings, and mind. This means that it must touch on gesture, emotion, and thought. It must also be perceived as a ritual of power by the sick person's ancestors, whether they reside on this or that side of the Great Threshold. It has to be a powerful ritual to face up to the information coming from the sick person's social and family system, cultural background, and above all imaginal tradition. The ritual has to impress, upset, shake, enchant.

There is undoubtedly a Western imaginal tradition and an Eastern imaginal tradition, and they differ. For someone belonging to the Tibetan Burmese Eng tribal group, living in a hut in the midst of the forest in Myanmar with an unaltered animist tradition going back to prehistoric times, a shamanic ritual centered on the sacrifice of a rooster, the beating of a drum, and ecstatic trance can be extremely effective. For a person with a Western imaginal tradition like ours, surgery can be a ritual capable of reestablishing the lost balance. That which is really important goes on inside the sick person and lies with the ability to turn a dramatic event into a ritual of sacrifice whereby the "I," the mind, may surrender, and the whole person may surrender to the mystery of invisibility, thus reestablishing the lost balance.

So it is not the cure itself that is effective but rather the way in which it is experienced. This explains why two people with the same illness and at the same stage, undergoing the same treatment, may face two differing prognoses.

The cure becomes rite at the moment of the ritual sacrifice, the *sacrum facere,* when the white bull (symbol of power) is returned to Poseidon (symbol of nature's divinity) by Minos (symbol of "I"), thus reestablishing the balance between human and nature.

If the rite is performed during the illness, the latter becomes the chance of a lifetime for the liberation of a human being. The same observations on illness can be applied to mental problems, emotional unrest, and, generally speaking, to life's troubles and problems.

2

The Great Image

THE MYSTICAL MARRIAGE

If everything in nature is beauty, is self-giving, so much so that things are impermanent, clear, and vivid dreams devoid of substance, if the system of images is so complex that everything is in the part and the part is in everything, if everything we observe in nature is, like a hologram or fractal, a complex image of which the smallest detail, observed under a microscope, shows the image of the whole, then nature is one image only, which repeats and repeats itself incessantly in infinite combinations. Consequently, delving deeper and deeper into each natural element—be it a blade of grass, a dew drop, the bark of a tree, a cricket, a thorn, an eagle, a rock, a mushroom, or the eye of a wolf—we should always, always come upon the same image.

This image, which can only be grasped by those who can see beyond appearances, beyond the deceit of the senses, beyond the hypnosis induced by the mind, is the Great Image.

This Great Image is the expression of the encounter between light and shadow, life and death. Every natural event is both living and dying, because all things that are born are already beginning to die in the instant of their birth. The living and the dying are always simultaneously present in every element of nature. Our body too, from the very moment of conception, begins to live, yet, at the same time, it begins to die.

The encounter of the dying with the living, of light with shadow, is the Great Image that lies in the depth of any and every natural image. This is an encounter of love, because it is a mutual and incessant self-giving. The dying gives itself to the living, and the living to the dying, light gives itself to shadow, and shadow to light, continuously. This self-giving underlies whatever we may possibly contemplate in nature.

We may also assert that this self-giving is the encounter of male with female, using these terms in their most ample meaning: male as in clarity, brightness, rationality, positivity, order, creation; female as in changeable, interiorizing, non-manifest, soul, emotional, vanishing. Let us finish with a poetic image, saying that only one and the same image underlies anything we may observe in nature, and it is the image of the encounter of love between the Mother and the Father.

The Great Image is the erotic union of the Mother and the Father; that is, a creative union. Creativity is one with self-giving, inasmuch as every creation implies a dying. In the erotic union of the Mother and the Father they give themselves to one another, dying, through their climax, the one in the body of the other.

Self-giving is creative pleasure, an annulment that implies ecstasy. This is why James Hillman declares in his book *The Dream and the Underworld* that "images love to vanish."

THE GREAT IMAGE IN
THE HEART OF RELIGIONS

All the religions in the world harbor two aspects: a revealed exoteric aspect and an initiatory and secret esoteric aspect. I should stress that the image of the erotic-creative union between the Mother and the

Father is amazingly shared by the heart of all religions.

I have traveled a lot due to both anthropological and naturalistic interests. Today I like to think that all the marvelous landscapes I have admired and all the people I have met have presented me with the same image of love, in multiple forms.

I went through my old travel logs and made a collage of the excerpts where I described my encounters with the Great Image. What follows is a short anthology of my geographic and inner journey, which bears witness to the existence of this powerful and universal image, which makes us all brothers and sisters.

THE GREAT IMAGE IN THE SHAMANIC YOGA TRADITION (SRI LANKA, 1985)

I first came into contact with the shamanic yoga tradition through Michael Williams. Through him I later made the acquaintance of extraordinary people such as the Sufi master Sheikh Salik, the renowned theologian Raimundo Panikkar, and the Maharaja Karan Singh . . . and it was thanks to Michael that I came into contact with the great Mother Mantra tradition that, from the very start, proved to be extraordinary.

The first wonder I witnessed was with Michael's own body.

At that time I had just turned nineteen. I was in Sri Lanka for work, for the first job of my life. I had been taken on by the Weligama Resort Hotel Ltd., a joint Italian Singhalese venture that was building a tourist village, a kind of oceanside paradise. My task was to take care of the bureaucracy and permits, standing in for the chairman when he was away. When in Weligama, where they were building the resort, I had an oceanside bungalow of my own. When I had to go to the capital, Colombo, for work errands I stayed at the Galadari Meridien Hotel, a big five-star hotel in a white tower opposite the old Parliament. After spending long and tiring days queuing in public offices, I would call Ratna, an ayurveda therapist, to the hotel and enjoy one of his extraordinary massages. Ratna was the owner of an ayurvedic massage school in Colombo. He was blind and was always accompanied by his assistant, a boy called Sarath.

I had told Ratna about myself, and he had understood that my life hadn't been easy, even though I was only nineteen, and that I suffered great inner torment. Whenever he could he insisted that I meet a certain Michael Williams, a great expert in yoga and shamanism and also an enlightened master endowed with *siddhis*; that is, yogic powers. At the time I couldn't tell the difference between yoga and yogurt; I was materialistic, and I had no idea that there might be something more useful to me than an ayurvedic massage. I kept on declining the offer to meet this teacher who I was told was more than sixty, and I imagined that he would be white-haired, full of wrinkles, slightly bent by age, veins bulging through the wrinkled skin on his forearms and legs, and with age-stained hands.

One day a waiter at the Galadari spilled my coffee. As he was preparing another one I realized that I was late for my massage, and I thought that Ratma and Sarath might already have been up to my room and, not seeing me there, might be searching for me. I got up to tell the waiter to forget about making me coffee and give me the bill, when I noticed Sarath. He was coming toward me, beaming. At the same time I noticed a tall, dark, slim man crossing the hotel hall. He was wearing a white straw hat; he was the most handsome male I had ever seen in my life. I watched him until he disappeared from my sight.

"Madam," said Sarath, "Ratma is waiting outside your room." I signed the bill and followed Sarath to the elevators. In the Galadari Meridien of Colombo there are two rows of elevators. The valet called us toward an elevator in the right row. I turned casually around and noticed the man with the white hat, who was waiting in the left row; my heart missed a beat and pearls of sweat broke out on my forehead. I promptly turned my back on him, nervously willing the elevator door to open.

Sarath touched my arm. "Do you remember the teacher of yoga and shamanism whom Ratma wants you to meet?" he asked. Without even giving me the chance to answer, he added, "He's right behind us." And that's how I made the acquaintance of the man who would decidedly change the course of my life.

Michael *was* more than sixty, but looked like he was under thirty. His body was lean, perfectly elastic, and harmonious; there was joy and enthusiasm in his eyes. He was an inspired man and had spent his life researching and practicing spirituality. One day, after our meeting, he told me a marvelous legend that he had been told by his teacher, who had been told it by *his* teacher. . . . Here is my description of the myth, told with the exact words written in my weathered diary from Sri Lanka, including the footnote.

The Legend of the Two Cougars

The legend of the two cougars always begins like this: "As long as life was sacred, self-giving, everything was joy and joy was everything."

Once, the world was populated only by couples of black and white cougars. In every couple, the white cougar and the black cougar loved each other and spent their time licking each other. The white cougar would lie between the paws of the black cougar, who would lick it and devour it. In turn, the white cougar would lick the black cougar from the inside and devour it. Then the white cougar would vomit the black one, re-creating it, and the whole cycle would begin over again. The two cougars feasted off each other incessantly and the light that glowed from the fire of their passion—which was the nectar of pleasure— generated couples of white and black cougars. One day, just as the white cougar was settling between the paws of the black cougar, there was an earthquake, which sent the white cougar rolling away from the black cougar. As the white cougar came near again, the black cougar noticed the fire of its own passion and found it wonderful. The black cougar fell in love with its own passion and devoured it.

When the white cougar came closer, the black cougar looked into its eyes and became frightened. Thinking that the white cougar wanted to devour it, the black cougar ran far, far away. Fearing that the white cougar might one day catch up with it, the black cougar began to create archers with the power derived from its union with the fire. The archers' task was to keep the white cougar at bay if it ever came close. They were born from fear, and so harbored the seed of evil. The archers began to build up a material world as a defense fort. Thus the world of matter and the objectivity of things was born. The black cougar lay down in the center of the material creation and, seeing itself surrounded only by night, fell asleep, and the fire inside it died out.

One day the white cougar found the black cougar and tried to get into the fort, but was kept away by the archers. Out of love, the white cougar tried several times to reach its beloved, until it decided to leap high over the world of matter, crossing it like a meteorite in its sky. The archers ripped open its belly with their arrows, and its heart was split in two by the point of an arrow and fell into the world, while its body passed away in the sky. The white cougar is now the king of the shadows, of the souls, of the invisible, of dreams, ancestors, of absence, of the unborn, of unaccomplished possibilities. Whereas the black cougar is the slumbering king of an existence that has become matter, evermore dense and heavy.

The two halves of the white cougar's heart represent two keys for the wakening from the hypnotic sleep that leads us to believe in the materialism and objectivity of things. One half has fallen into this world, the other half has sunk into the underworld. *

---

*Note: Michael called the half-heart in the underworld the Mother Key and the half-heart in this world the Father Key. The broken heart of the cougar testifies that the path to awakening is to be walked both on this side and that side of the Great Threshold, in life as in death, in day as in night, in light as in darkness.

THE GREAT IMAGE IN
THE ESOTERIC CHRISTIAN TRADITION
(SWITZERLAND, 2003)

In 2003 a great scholar of alchemy, Paolo Lucarelli, helped me to stage a convention at Campione d'Italia. That year we managed to create a highly mystical and spiritual event near the biggest casino of Europe, in the Italian Las Vegas, in a country famous for its gambling.

Many illustrious scholars took part in the convention, including James Hillman, whom I consider my Western teacher, several learned esoteric exponents, and renowned philosophers and academics. It was a unique opportunity for me to delve deeper into the topic of Gnosticism.

Here are the notes from my diary.

Christian Gnosticism

Christian Gnosticism is a current of ancient Christianity, which developed in Alexandria of Egypt under the influence of Neo-Platonism. Gnosticism is a syncretic religion that reunites pre-Christian religions and philosophies with the original Christianity, founded on the so-called gnostic gospels, the Apocrypha, like the well-known Gospel of Judas.

The Apocrypha

The term apocryphal *means "to be hidden," "reserved for few." The Apocrypha are spiritual scriptures that refer to the figure of Jesus. Unlike the standard gospels, these scriptures were not accepted as official by the church, and were not included in the Christian canon. They were destroyed and lost, only a few fragments having reached us. Their destruction points to evidence that they were most likely considered "bothersome" for the empire. It is indeed said that when the emperor Constantine decided to unify his empire with the Christian religion, spreading its vision to unite all the populations under his domain, and preferring the standard gospels to the more "bothersome" apocryphal ones, he had the latter destroyed.*

Yet Gnosticism continued to grow in Western mystic cults and doctrines, such as alchemy. Gnosticism has weaved its way through the history of Western philosophical and mystic thinking, surfacing in several movements that refer to it more or less openly, such as in Theosophy, and the writings of C. G. Jung and James Hillman.

Sophia

According to the Gnostics, God is both male and female.

The paradise of the Gnostics, the Pleroma, is inhabited by couples of Aeons, always made up of a male and a female Aeon. The Aeons are emanated from a Primal Aeon God or Monad or Perfect Aeon, which is both Mother and Father.

In its last emanation, the Primal Aeon emanates the Soter Aeon and the Sophia Aeon. The female Aeon, Sophia, causes instability in the Pleroma because it creates without its male counterpart, Soter, the Christ, giving rise to the tragic Demiurge Yahweh, Satan, the violent Old Testament God, which in turn gives rise to the formerly inexistent world of matter.

It is a dark, heavy world, a fallen world. The so-called Archons emanate from Yahweh, with the task of bringing the dark world of matter back to the divine Pleroma. But the tools they use to do so are laws, rules, and regulations. So instead of bringing the dark world closer, the Archons move it further away from the Pleroma.

The Gnostic myth tells of the universe's drama whereby, even though the universe struggles to adhere to the criteria of good and bad created by reason, even though it forces itself to follow the rules dictated by logos, it develops a technocratic civilization that cannot stop the destruction of nature and, dismayed, witnesses the continuous deforestation of the planet and the ongoing disappearance of living species.

Salvation cannot only be in the mind.

The Aeon called Sophia, realizing what has happened, leaps into the material world, becoming the spark of light within each and every creature, thanks to which they may make their way back to the divine Pleroma. Then Sophia takes on human form as Mary Magdalen. The Christ, too, takes on human form to teach humans the way back to the Pleroma, the gnosis.

The word gnosis *means "knowledge." It is an enlightened knowledge that may be reached through a personal journey in the search for truth. This obviously makes Gnosticism a heretic movement according to the orthodox church, which preaches the observance of the cult and canonic precepts.*

The Gnostic way is said to have been taught by the Christ to a handful of disciples in the time between the Resurrection and the Ascension, which, according to the Gnostics, lasted eleven years, not just forty days. The apocryphal gospel Pistis Sophia is about this teaching, which was apparently handed down by occult factions within the Christian institutions for the benefit of the elected few, and excluding the ecclesiastic hierarchy.

The first great teacher of the Christ's teachings is said to have been the Magdalen herself, who is described as the bride and priestess of Jesus, symbol of the gnosis. According to several occult factions, Jesus invested the Magdalen with the responsibility of spreading the doctrine. Jesus is said to have had at least one child from the Magdalen.

In his use of the Christian religion as a tool for unifying his empire with a common system of values and beliefs, the emperor Constantine allegedly kept only four gospels, the most harmless and most useful, and ordered the destruction of the others; he also allegedly substituted the figure of the Magdalen with that of Peter and Paul. It would have been inconceivable for a woman to act as the keeper of the faith on which an empire with a patriarch-centered model of reality was to be founded. Constantine is also said to have ordered the elimination of the Christ's descendants. This was left unaccomplished though, because the keepers of the Sang Real, symbolically the Holy Grail, sought refuge in France where they were allegedly protected by the legendary, invincible Knights Templars. From France the guardians of the Holy Grail then moved on to Scotland, where they apparently founded esoteric factions for passing down the secrets. One of the most mysterious and suggestive places today is the Roslyn Chapel near Edinburgh, where the gnostic secrets are said to be kept.

THE GREAT IMAGE
IN ESOTERIC BUDDHISM
(BHUTAN, 1996)

Here are some notes I jotted down in my diary when I traveled to Bhutan. I organized this trip to Bhutan with the help of Adri Drolma Shama, an extraordinary woman whom I met thanks to an important Swiss tour operator. Adri Drolma Shama is an anthropologist and wife of a minister of His Majesty Jigme Singye Wangchuck, fourth king of Bhutan.

Discovering the Vajradhara (May 27, 1996)

In Bhutan, in certain sacred places, I found an extraordinary image: the Vajradhara, a magnificent representation of non-duality, in which the Buddha is represented in erotic intercourse with his partner. This is the primordial Buddha, the central symbol of esoteric Buddhism, also known as Vajrayana Buddhism or tantric Buddhism. Bhutan, which has always been isolated by the imposing Himalayan mountain chain, is the only country today that still considers tantric Buddhism the official religion. For the tantric disciple the Vajradhara is the essence of Buddhism, embodied in Buddha Shakyamuni, who is an emanation of enlightenment, whereas Vajradhana is the very light of enlightenment. Here in Bhutan these forms are considered so tremendously powerful that spontaneous liberation is deemed possible by simply contemplating them.

Some of the marvelous effigies of the Vajradhara in Bhutan express the peaceful form of the divinity, whereas other more interesting ones express the many angry forms. The angry form is more powerful than the peaceful form and bestows more intense visions and powers, but the ability to embody and represent it is the result of a long and complex spiritual journey.

The Flying Monks (June 11, 1996)

Thanks to Adri Drolma Shama I came into contact with a group of Buddhist monks, followers of the Divine Madman. Drukpa Kunliley, a.k.a. the Divine Yogin Madman, is one of the most venerated saints in Bhutan. He preached the desecration of religious and lay institutions—convinced they were the main obstructions to awakening—through eroticism and exhilaration, both effective paths to spiritual enlightenment. The core method was kept secret and passed on to very few to avoid a mainstream misunderstanding.

The monastery of the so-called flying monks is perched high on a steep cliff in the middle of the Black Mountain National Park, where the black-necked cranes come to rest after their migration from Siberia and Tibet. My friend told me that in this monastery, the followers of the Divine Madman embody the angry form of the Great Mother. This is accomplished through a ritual whereby the monks run along the high, narrow walls of the monastery, covered by a jute sack so that they can't see, guided only by the screeching of the eagles and their spiritual eye, which is drawn on the jute sack at groin level. After this extraordinary ritual, the monks become oracles, messengers of the Great Mother, and capable of predicting the future.

In the monastery of the flying monks, I spent the whole day talking with the lama guardian. He taught me a meditation method. He told me to meditate on the image of the Vajradhara seated in the position of erotic intercourse with his partner. He gave me precise indications of visualizing the Buddha with the color blue above his head, on the mystic point that is 9 inches above his head and 9 inches in front of his forehead. Then he told me to visualize a Vajradhara with the color red at the heart center. As we will see, it is extraordinary how the lama's instructions coincide with the teachings regarding the tradition of the mystical marriage!

THE GREAT IMAGE IN THE ANIMIST TRADITION

Between 1990 and 2003, I did a lot of traveling. I visited several animist tribes in Asia and South America, motivated by the desire to learn more about shamanism, which Michael's teachings had endeared me to. Here are some brief notes from that period.

The Animist Akha
(September 9, 1999)

Animism is the ancient religion of the Great Mother, which is born from a deep contact with the soul of the world. For the animist populations, every aspect of nature has a soul. Our predecessors were certainly animists: animism is the religion of the prehistoric peoples.

Today, animist populations are scattered throughout the forests of Asia. The Akha are the most numerous. At both entrances to their villages you often see a sacred bamboo gate in honor of the protecting spirits of the community. At one side of the gate is a wooden circle with a hole in the middle, to symbolize the female essence; at the other side of the gate a vertical trunk with a single knob represents the male essence; tied to the gate is a very long chain of bamboo rings, one for every tribal ancestor.

Spirits of Nature
(February 2, 2002)

In the forests of Myanmar live Burmese shamans who still worship the Nat, the spirits of nature, and still celebrate Nat Kadow, the rite of matrimony between human and Nat.

Today Wai Lan Lan, a shaman who lives on the plain of Pagan, the "city of pagans," as it was called by the English colonists, told me her story. She has two husbands, an earthly one and a celestial one. She has a son of flesh and blood from her earthly husband, and from her celestial husband she has many invisible children, which are her most creative ideas and her most melodious songs. Indeed Wai Lan Lan sings in an orchestral choir, which plays Burmese music. Every Friday evening the shaman leaves her husband and son at home and goes back to the village of her childhood to sleep with her celestial husband, one of the 37 Nat, spirits or lords of nature, who rule the pantheon of Burmese animism. This particular Nat passes on to Wai Lan Lan its shamanic powers, which she uses for the benefit of the people of Pagan. They are mostly mediumistic powers. When someone comes to Wai Lan Lan with a problem, she falls into a shamanic trance with the help of her celestial husband, who ferries her to the otherworld, and when she returns she brings back a solution, a remedy, or some advice.

FURTHER CONSIDERATIONS ON THE GREAT IMAGE (SWITZERLAND, 2003)

I jotted down the following notes in my diary in 2003, the year of the previously mentioned convention at Campione d'Italia. I can't remember whether before or after.

Hinduism

In Hinduism there are several pairs of divinities, couples who are inseparable from each other. They symbolize the non-duality of the opposites, which are distinct but not separate. Shiva is the erotic ascetic inseparable from Parvathi, who is his Shakti, his own force. When he takes to lone meditation and to leading an ascetic life in the forest, he is nevertheless united to Parvathi through his tapas, *his asceticism and self-discipline. The word* tapas *literally means "fire," which can indicate both spiritual ardor and the fire of passion (*kama*) for Parvathi. By the means of this fire, Shiva works all kinds of magical wonders, including burning the worlds and regenerating them.*

Rama and Sita are another couple of Hindu divinities who symbolize the mystic union.

The Alchemists and Rosy Cross

The Great Image is the secret ingredient of the alchemists, the catalyst that allows the Rubedo, or the Opus in Red, by which matter, after evaporating, turns into pure gold.

Alchemy is an ancient esoteric philosophical system that has intrigued many scholars over the centuries, among them the great C. G. Jung and several post-Jungians, including James Hillman. The whole branch of deep psychology, which sparked from Jung, is deeply nurtured by the occult knowledge of alchemy.

The Great Opus of the alchemist is a coniunctio oppositorum *(conjunction of opposites) in which silver and gold, the moon and the sun, shadow and light, male and female, unite. The alchemic transmutation, by purifying matter with fire, brings it back to its true nature, which is image, and at the same time frees the alchemist from the idea that that which glitters is not gold, enabling the hieratic wedding, the sacred matrimony, between all the opposites.*

The Chymical Wedding of Christian Rosenkreuz (Rosy Cross) *is the title of a romance generally attributed to Johann Valentin Andreae; it is considered one of the manifestos of the Rosicrucian brotherhood. Many poets and alchemists have been inspired by this romance over the epochs, the mystical marriage being the aim of alchemy.*

In the romance Christian Rosenkreuz is invited to a magic castle for the sacred wedding of a king and a queen. In actual fact it is the account of an initiation with its rituals of death and rebirth, purification and resurrection. The plot of the Chymical Wedding *is set 150 years before its publication and begins on Easter Day 1459; that is, on the same day that the constitutive act of the Strasbourg Freemasonry was signed.*

No one knows whether Christian Rosenkreuz ever existed, or whether he is an allegorical figure. Rudolf Steiner, an Austrian philosopher, social reformer, and founder of the esoteric and spiritual movement named anthroposophy, among others, identified him as diverse initiates throughout history, as though he were the recurring spirit of a master. Indeed, in the works attributed to him, many journeys are undertaken to the East to increase his occult, mystical, and gnostic knowledge.

His name, too—Christian Rosenkreuz, or "Rosy Cross"— testifies openly that there are two forms of Christianity: just as there are two streams in all the religions of the world, so in Christianity there is a mainstream determined and preached by the ecclesiastic hierarchy, and another occult, secret faction whose knowledge is passed on through other, non-canonical environments, without involving the hierarchy.

Christian Mysticism

The history of Christian mysticism is brimming with examples of alchemical union between the Divine and the human. I came upon an extraordinary booklet titled O Dulcissime Amplexator, *written by Hildegard von Bingen, a twelfth-century German nun. Hildegard is one of the most striking and fascinating people of her time, with interests ranging from theology, to art, biology, herbs, dramaturgy, and music. Summing up, she was an artist, herbalist, and sorceress; she founded a monastic community, which still lives on today. She led an eventful life, punctuated by celestial visions in which, as is true of her lyrics, carnal love unites with divine love to generate something absolutely unique. Hildegard's very original interpretation of monastic virginity as a symbol of a more authentic, sublime, and total carnal passion earned her much criticism when, at certain feasts, she allowed nuns to dance, wearing special clothes and crowns to state their virginity. Hildegard's model for her songs and music were the Gregorian chants that, to our day, fascinate and uplift the listener.*

With her own Gregorian chants, Hildegard von Bingen gives us a moving example of a mystical marriage, among other more renowned examples coming from the history of Christian mysticism, such as Saint Teresa of Avila, or Saint Clare, and Saint Francis.

Here are the lyrics to one of my favorite songs of hers.

Symphonia Virginum*

Oh lover sweet,
so sweet the embrace:
Help us to keep
our virginity!
[. . .]
Now unto you we crym our bridegroom and our
*   consolation*
[. . .]
For in your blood we are betrothed to you—
your blood our wedding gift;
for mortal husbands we refuse, choosing you instead,
the Son of God.

O beauteous form, O fragrance sweeter than
the most desired of delights:
our sighs of longing ever seek for you

---

*Latin collated from the transcription of Beverly Lomer and the edition of Barbara Newman; translation by Nathaniel M. Campbell, www.hildegard-society .org/2017/05/o-dulcissime-amator-symphonia-virginum.html.

within this lonely wilderness of tears.
When shall we look on you
and with you ever stay?

We live within the world,
and you within our minds,
and we embrace you in our hearts
as if you're present even now.

The mighty lion, you have burst the heavens,
descending to the Virgin's palace-womb,
destroying death
and building life within a golden city.

Grant us her company
to dwell with you, O bridegroom sweet,
who saved us from the devil's jaws
who dragged our primal parents into death.

THE GREAT IMAGE IN ISLAM
(YEMEN, 1993)

I have traveled extensively in Yemen thanks to the extraordinary friendship of Sheikh Salik, an Imam (a spiritual guide of an Islamic Sufi community). Sufism is a creative, spiritual, and non-doctrinal blend of Islam, esotericism, magic, and alchemy. The Sufis are the mystics of Islam and have not always been well regarded by orthodox Islam; indeed they have even been persecuted for heresy, which seems to be the common destiny for many true mystics in the history of humanity, regardless of their religious tradition.

Sheikh Salik was the leader of the Sufi Alwan order, which is inspired by the works and life of the great poet Ahamed bin Alwan. I was introduced to Sheikh Salik by Michael Williams, my yoga teacher.

Without this introduction I would have stood a very slim chance of connecting with the Yemenite Sufis, because they lead a very reserved life and their cults, practices, and meetings are kept secret. They dislike opening up to the outside, and they especially dislike revealing themselves to non-Muslims.

The Hadra

Thanks to the generosity of Sheikh Salik, I was allowed to witness the hadra, Sufi rituals based on mystic ecstasy. The hadra are the ceremonies where the dervishes go into a trance, accompanied by the beating of drums, dancing, and singing. Of all the magnificent reunions I witnessed, one in particular struck me, in a mosque in the middle of the desert.

Before going to the desert, I asked Sheikh Salik about the rite. He explained that according to the Sufi vision, human beings are made of sand and soul. Everything in this world has a double nature, and even Allah needs to have a counterpart to enter this world. The Sufi rite is the sacrifice of Allah who dies, separating from the sand, leaving the earthly world to return to the celestial world. The Imam went on, "So, during the Sufi rite, we die and our souls abandon our bodies and rise to the skies. There they receive nourishment and then return to the sand, allowing us to be reborn. Through death and rebirth our eyes open, our minds see, our bodies heal." He added, "There are one hundred and twenty-four thousand eyes in the body and in the earth, and the biggest eye of the earth is the sky."

After this introduction, I, along with two Swiss women traveling with me and our interpreter guide Alì, followed the Imam to the mosque.

Darkness was about to give way to night when suddenly an extraordinary full moon, so big it seemed one could simply reach out and touch it, rose quickly on the horizon, from behind the sand dunes. The moonlight gave an eerie silvery fluorescence to the walls of the mosque.

Then, in a flash, like bullets in the moonlight, a multitude of jeeps appeared from behind the dunes out of nowhere with a muffled and distant buzz; like a swarm of bees rushing from the hive, they closed in on the mosque.

Ten, twenty, fifty, a hundred . . . it seemed they were never-ending.

The jeeps parked near the mosque, and many men—actually only men, not even one woman—clambered out. They were wearing the Yemenite ritual costume with the thick belt and proper sheath for the jambee, the typical Yemenite dagger. Several had rifles slung from their shoulders, others carried drums, and most had a lopsided swelling of one cheek from their habit of keeping a bolus of qat grass in their mouths. (Qat is a local plant that, similar to cocaine leaves, acts like a stimulant. Qat releases its stimulating substance on contact with the saliva, which is why it is chewed into a bolus and kept between the teeth and the cheek for a long time.)

Sheikh Salik was all dressed in white, and his head was covered by a white veil that shimmered in the moonlight. All around us hundreds of men greeted and hugged each other. "You will have to stay here while we enter the mosque for the first part of the ritual, and then we shall perform the second part outside for you, as promised," said the interpreter, translating the words of Sheikh Salik.

At that moment two men passed us by, carrying a man who could not walk so that only the tips of his toes dragged over the ground, leaving two furrows in the sand. "He is ill," explained the Imam, "and he is here in the hope that the energy of the hadra may help to heal him."

We did as Sheikh told us, and waited outside the mosque, chatting and admiring the moon. The Sufis came out of the mosque after less than an hour, following Sheikh Salik. They all sat down in a big circle under the fluorescent wall of the mosque. Our interpreter asked us to sit nearby and stayed with us.

The Sufis started to beat the drums and chant the name of Allah in a crescendo, in unison of voice and breath, quickly becoming a very loud, primordial "Ah, Ah, Ah, Ah . . ."

We three women had never felt such a powerful energy in such a crescendo. Indeed it was an energy that could have quickened the dead.

Throughout the hadra, the Sheikh was in a trance and his eyes were upturned to the whites, his pupils invisible, like a dead man. Yet he was the one who chanted and breathed most vigorously, his body continuously swaying back and forth rhythmically. During this deep breathing mens' abdomens were contracted in the moment of exhalation, giving tremendous strength to the breath. All that energy was channeled through a bowl of fresh water that was in the center of this incredible circle of men.

At the end of the ceremony, the Sheikh came and hugged us good-bye, as though we were not in a Muslim country, as though we were not from this world, and said, "That which is not in a hadra, is nowhere to be found. What you receive from a hadra will stay with you forever. From ceremony to ceremony, the soul is restored at the source of love, and becomes ever stronger, able to withstand the ecstasy of pleasure."

All the great Sufi masters are poets and have always sung their love of God, passionate, carnal, and physical love, as is also expressed in the Song of Songs (or Canticle of Canticles) in the Bible.

Here are some verses from the great Rumi, considered the founder of the Sufis.

> *I need a lover who,*
> *every time he awakes,*
> *gives rise to infinite worlds of fire*
> *from every part of the world!*
> *I want a heart like hell,*
> *which breathes the fire of hell,*
> *churning two hundred seas,*
> *the waves withstanding!*
> *A lover who wraps the skies*

like linen around his hands
and hangs the candle of eternity
like a chandelier,
enters into battle like a lion
with the valor of Leviathan,
leaves nothing but himself
then fights with himself, too,
and, tearing away the seven hundred veils
from his heart with his light,
may the crying call descend on the world
from his high throne;
and when, from the seventh sea,
he turns to the mysterious mounts of Qaf,
from that far ocean will spread pearls from the dust.

MORE POETRY

In every population's spiritual tradition there are many examples of visionary songs and poems that offer praise to the mystical marriage. Let us take as example "The Canticle of Canticles," the marvelous hymn inserted in the Bible by will of the faithful, becoming part of the Christian canon.

Following is a selection of verses (from the Douay-Rheims Bible translation).

Put me as a seal upon thy heart,
as a seal upon thy arm,
for love is strong as death,
 jealousy as hard as hell,
the lamps thereof are fire and flames.
Many waters cannot quench charity,
neither can the floods drown it. (8:6–7)

Let him kiss me with the kiss of his mouth:
for thy breasts are better than wine,
Smelling sweet of the best ointments.
Thy name is as oil poured out:
therefore young maidens have loved thee.
Draw me: we will run after thee
to the odor of thy ointments.
The king hath brought me into his storerooms:
we will be glad and rejoice in thee,
remembering thy breasts more than wine:
the righteous love thee. (1:2–3)

In my bed by night I sought him
whom my soul loveth:
I sought him, and found him not.
I will rise, and will go about the city:
in the streets and the broad ways
I will seek him whom my soul loveth:
I sought him, and I found him not.
The watchmen who keep the city, found me:
Have you seen him, whom my soul loveth?
When I had a little passed by them,
I found him whom my soul loveth:
I held him: and I will not let him go,
till I bring him into my mother's house,
and into the chamber of her that bore me. (3:1–4)

The words are imbued with sacredness. The Christian readers of the canticle have often allegorized or spiritualized it, offended by its physical exuberance. Yet the canticle *is* very physical: here love happens in nature, without ever, not even for a single instant, forgetting its sacred essence.

3

The Underworld
or Celestial Bride/
Bridegroom

IF THE MYSTICAL MARRIAGE IS ACTUALLY CELEBRATED, it isn't some faraway event in heaven. It happens inside every one of us, daily. The more intensely we are aware of our union with our underworld or celestial bride/bridegroom, the stronger is our energy, the more abundant is our inspiration, and the more joyful is our existence.

It's a question of awareness.

The Father and the Mother united in the ecstasy of passion are the two aspects of ourselves: us and our soul. The male aspect is our mind, our visible aspect: the living being that is on this side of the Great Threshold, in the time-space dimension. The female aspect is our shadow, our invisible aspect: the dying being beyond the Great Threshold who is passing from death to the next birth, not in the space-time dimension.

In the tradition of teachings about after-death experiences, as represented in the *Bardo Tosgrol,* the Tibetan Book of the Dead, the living is shrouded in a body of flesh and blood, which is either the result of accumulated karma (action) or, for the enlightened, is chosen at the moment of conception. The dying, on the other hand, resides in the body of *bardo*. The word *bardo* means "transit," in this case meaning the transit from death to birth. The body of bardo is endowed with all the senses, and, like the body of flesh and blood, it can see, hear, touch, smell, and taste, but it is invisible and may travel at the speed of thought.

The body of bardo and the body of flesh and blood are simultaneous, inasmuch as both started living at the moment of conception, and, at that very same moment, both started dying. The living and the dying are within each other, joined in a permanent erotic-creative bond.

Our "I," finite in itself and separated from everything, is an abstract, illusionary principle that imprisons and limits us. But our "I," united with our soul, the invisible part of us, our shadow, which lives beyond the Great Threshold, is a principle of pure non-dual awareness that may lead us to the final liberation.

Our mystical bridegroom/bride is not external to us; it is not other, it is the invisible part of us that is projected into the world. It is our soul, and it is the *anima mundi* (world soul), the invisible aspect of every thing, every person, every place.

THE IMMOVABLE PLEASURE

Every one of us is permanently joined to the anima mundi through an erotic-creative relationship; this state is defined as "immovable pleasure" in alchemy and in the shamanic-tantric yoga tradition. Immovable pleasure is a state of pervasive excitement; that is, of constant creativity and inspiration that never slips away, because it is independent of any external object.

Immovable pleasure is independent of any external object, because it can only be reached through the awakening of awareness, which enables us to see the illusionary state of all material objects. This awakened awareness, understanding the void essence of every thing, begins to relate to the soul of things; that is, to their invisible aspect, which it perceives beyond that which the eyes can behold.

To be in a state of immovable pleasure means to be in a similar state to those moments of ecstatic trance when a shaman communicates with the spirits. In this state—which is the condition of the alchemical wedding—it is possible to talk to the swarms of spirits, demons, deities, and genies who populate the invisible, empty universe. They are the infinite aspects of our soul—the lords of nature, the natural forces that in a certain esoteric tradition are called by names such as gnomes (the spirits of the earth), undines (the spirits of the waters), salamanders (the spirits of the fire), and sylphs (the spirits of the air). They are our ideas; they are our ancestors, who are not absent but invisible. They are our wild soul, our animal spirit, and our subtle guides, our inner teacher. They are the *elohim,* the extraterrestrial beings who, according to some, are supposed to have shaped the human race. These are all aspects of our mystical bridegroom/bride, because—as we said—the soul is of such complexity that everything is in the part and the part is in everything, the multiple in one and one in the multiple.

Our underworld or celestial bride/bridegroom is always around us and embraces us. We are permanently joined to the invisible in an erotic-creative union.

EROS, THE CREATIVE ENERGY

As James Hillman used to say, Hades is also Dionysus: "There is a dance in death. Hades and Dionysus are the same."* Hades is Dionysus, the personification of the erotic, irrational, and wild force of nature. Hillman also clarified: "Eros is the brother of death and not the principle that will save us from it. . . . Thus there is a downward

---

*James Hillman, *The Dream and the Underworld* (New York: HarperCollins, 1979), 33.

love, and not only an Eros stretching its arms towards the horizons."*

Hades is also Zeus, because, in a complex universe, the high and the low reflect each other; that is, to state one of the hermetic principles: As above, so below. Hades also corresponds to Persephone, his bride, the queen of the underworld.

Our partner in the mystical marriage may be either male or female, depending on what mainly moves our set of erotic images. The underworld partner must be imagined in the manners and forms that most stimulate our erotic imagination, because true knowledge is triggered by the creative force, Eros.

NONDISPERSION OF THE JUICE OF PLEASURE

Each one of us is permanently in an erotic-creative union with an invisible bridegroom/bride in whose body we incessantly die and from whose body we are incessantly born. It is an orgasmic relationship of which the genital aspect is only a reflex, a reminder, a representation.

Our true erotic relationship is with the king, or queen, of the invisible. Our invisible partner is many in one and one in many, so our partner is ours exclusively, yet at the same time is as many as there are men and women in the world.

The genital aspect, which is commonly experienced with our earthly partner, the individual, acts as a reminder of our divine union. When the divine union is fully accomplished, the reminder is no longer needed.

Tantric yoga and alchemy—which are the guiding paths in the mystical marriage—teach that one should never disperse the juices of male and female pleasure. In tantrism it is even said that "the juice of pleasure must flow back up to melt a pearl of light (called Tig Le), which will drip the sweetness of the deities' juice into the body." In the genital

*James Hillman, *The Dream and the Underworld*, 48.

act, which symbolizes the divine union, the semen is dispersed when it is not used for procreation. Equally, in the divine union, semen is dispersed when it is not used for creation.

To be in a permanent state of immovable pleasure, in constant union with the invisible partner, it is mandatory to remain in constant creativity, which is pleasure, never accepting or allowing oneself to be convinced to carry out non-creative unpleasurable actions.

When the body lacks inner pleasure it enters into a state of contrition; when consciousness lacks pleasure it becomes dimmed; when the mind lacks pleasure it becomes cold and isolated. In this unfavorable state of affairs one becomes trapped in the wheel of illusions, and the reawakening is kept at bay. So it is very important to maintain pleasure in the body, in awareness, in the mind.

Creative pleasure is a fire, which in tantric-shamanic yoga is called *dumo* or *tumo* in Tibet and *tapas* in India. Tapas is the omnipresent fire, kindled in those who are in the mystical marriage with divinity and who have surpassed the genital dimension, which often leads to the dispersion of semen. It is an animistic fire born in the belly, two fingers below the belly button; it then is kindled and flares upward. In the highest creative moments it may spread to the seventh chakra at the summit of the head, where the fontanelle is found, and even beyond, up to the mystical point a hand's span above the head. The masters say that the animistic fire should never be allowed to die down. To avoid this happening, human beings should always lead a creative life, avoiding unpleasurable routine actions.

THE SEPARATION OF THE DIVINE LOVERS

A human being who is fully aware of union with the celestial or underworld bride/bridegroom is free. Such a man is free because his bride is his teacher, his only guide. Such a woman is free because her bridegroom is her immeasurable pleasure, and she is fulfilled; she needs nothing else. Such a person has the favor of the gods and has been elected to freedom, going beyond good and evil. In the beauty of the natural state such a person doesn't reason in terms of personal advantage or disadvantage so cannot be manipulated.

Freedom is not suited to the need for control, for the "I's" will for power. For the "I" to keep its illusion of power and control over nature, over the body, over emotions, over the soul, it thinks in such a manner as to separate the divine lovers on the one hand and confirm the genital experience as the source of pleasure on the other. Our world is founded on these two operations, these two pillars. If only one is demolished, the whole world falls apart.

The Separation of the Divine Lovers in the Macrocosmos

Important repercussions ensue from the psychological process, the illusion of the separation of the divine lovers. This manifests in a macrocosmic manner by the extraction of the Father from the Mother's body, putting an end to the cosmic orgasm, the immovable pleasure. The Father, separated from the Mother, is then taken up and set in a far sky to become metaphysical, vouching for the values of good and bad on which civilization is founded.

The Mother, nature, deprived of her spirit, the Father, sinks into the heaviness of materialism, becoming object. The female dimension thus becomes an object of matter to be exploited, whereas the spirit lives in some faraway sky.

In Inca mythology there is a legend that marvelously explains the birth, evolution, and overcoming of this metaphysical vision that is the pillar of materialistic deception.

It is said that Pachacamac, the sky, fertilized the earth, Pachamama, with its semen, the rain. Two twins were born from this union, a boy and a girl.

Then Pachacamac, the god of the sky, fell under the spell of an evil magician, Wakon, who wanted to possess Mother Earth.

In a dark world with no sky, Pachamama was left alone to fight all kinds of monsters with her two children, as they attempted to reach a feeble, faraway light.

One day they finally managed to reach the light. It came from the cave of Wakon, who was expecting them. Wakon said he wanted to cook a potato in a big stone cauldron. He asked the children to go and fetch some water.

As soon as the children set off, Wakon tried to seduce Pachamama, but to no avail. So Wakon killed and devoured Pachamama, hiding her remains in the cauldron. But Pachacamac, being immortal, was still alive, and sent a new dawn after the long night on earth.

Huaychau, the bird who was to announce daybreak, caught Wakon with his mouth still dripping blood; he took pity on the two children, telling them what had happened to their mother, and warning them of the danger they risked by staying with Wakon. So the children ran away while Wakon was asleep.

On their way, the twins met a fox, Anas, who hid them in its den after hearing their story. In the meantime Wakon had woken up and was looking for them. First he asked all the animals he met if they had seen the children, but none of them helped him because all the wild animals were helping the children in their escape. Then he met Anas. The fox tricked him by saying that the children were on top of a mountain and that he could catch them by imitating their mother's voice when he got to the mountaintop.

Wakon ran off toward the mountaintop with a puff and a pant but fell into a deep hole that the fox had hidden by covering it up with a thin layer of sticks and leaves. Wakon was killed in the fall, causing a violent earthquake.

Freed of the dangerous Wakon, the twins were brought up by Anas and nurtured with Anas's own blood. One day they saw a rope dangling from the sky. They were curious and climbed up. At the top Pachacamac was waiting for them and rewarded them by turning the boy into the sun and the girl into the moon.

As for Pachamama, she stayed below forever, taking on the form of a great snowfield, still called La Viuda (the widow).

In the "I," and in the world, there is a will (Wakon), which strives to dominate and possess nature (Pachamama) and ends up raping and devouring her. But salvation is always feasible for human beings who strive for freedom instead.

The Separation of the Divine Lovers in the Microcosmos

The illusion of the division between *res cogitans* (thinking substance) and *res extensa* (material substance) leads us to live as though our body is an object, losing the awareness of its symbolic value; this turns us into eco-incompatible individuals.

Water, air, earth, and fire are emotions and experiences that meet in the pleasure of sameness.

Earth is the experience of softness and hardness, of heaviness and levity.

Water is the experience of dryness and wetness.

Fire is the experience of heat and cold.

Air is the experience of movement and stillness.

These experiences bring forth emotions of contact, being born from the impact between the visible and the invisible, between light and shadow. The variations in intensity and quality are potentially infinite. They represent the sensations that can be felt in the erotic-creative love relationship.

The separation of matter from spirit turns the elements into objects and forces the subject perceiving them to succumb to their impact. The objectification of reality—the separation of the object that is experienced from the object that is experiencing—leads the individual to lose contact with the soul, which is in itself the act of imagining and creating out of love.

THE SOUL AND ITS MISSION

The soul gives rise to the experiences of earth, water, fire, and air by imagining the beauty of self-giving: love, vanishing for love, and creating for love. Imagining means creating for love. In depth psychology the terms *psyche, soul,* and *instinct* are often considered synonyms, used to define the creative activity that generates all the impressions we inhabit. This creative imagining solely regards the aspect of the contact between Mother and Father, death and life, light and shadow.

The deceptive perception of the separation of the divine lovers makes us lose contact with the imaginal. Losing touch with the imaginal, we forget that we are the projectors of the images that we inhabit. And like the dreamers of a dream, having forgotten that we are in a dream, we succumb to the events and to the impact with the elements, which are images we have wrought ourselves.

The awakening from the dream is when the divine lovers are reunited and immovable pleasure is reestablished.

THE SOUL'S MISSION

The soul comes into the world with a mission based on the need to activate certain behavior patterns, and to do so it uses certain original images, or archetypes. What we now call *archetypes* in today's depth psychology were once known as gods, or spirits by the shamans and animistic populations. They are the original forms of experience.

For a behavior pattern to manifest in the world it is undoubtedly necessary for it first to be imagined somehow. Nothing that has not been imagined beforehand can happen. For example, if instinct had not imagined the hunt, the forging of the first arrow, and the killing of the first mammoth, then those behaviors would not have manifested, and perhaps there would only be vegetarians on this planet. That which is the spirit of the hunt for the shaman is the archetype of the hunt for the psychologist, while in ancient Greece it was Artemis, the goddess of the hunt.

The main images our soul projects, like the gods in a myth, bring about events and tales of passion, of magnificent and beautiful unrest, beyond good and evil. These tales are our lives. This is what brought James Hillman to say, "We can only do in time what the gods do in eternity."*

The process of reabsorption of reality, which may be accomplished through the methods of the Mother Mantra tradition, enables us to witness the myth that we are enacting and living on the scene of life. The awareness of the myth that we are involved in allows us to become lovers, partners, accomplices of the gods, relieving us from feeling that we are victims of events. James Hillman recalls us to the message of Hades.

> Hades is the final cause, the aim, the telos of every soul and of every animistic process.
>
> Where is my destiny, my process of individualization, taking me? If we are honest enough to answer this question, the answer is staring at us: the process of individualization is leading us to death. This unfathomable destination is the only absolutely certain event of the human condition. Hades is the invisible, yet it is always with us. The divine call to Hades implies that all the

*James Hillman, *The Vain Escape from the Gods* (Thompson, Conn.: Spring Publications, 1989), 21.

aspects of the ongoing soul are to be treated bearing in mind the end.*

The mission of the soul is to give itself. It is love; it is beauty and the beauty of pleasure, all expressions of love. It is for this end that the soul manifests all the images, which is why images love to vanish.

---

*James Hillman, *The Dream and the Underworld* (New York: HarperCollins, 1979), 44, 45.

4

The Four Movements of the Mother Mantra Tradition

THE FUNCTION OF THE MOTHER MANTRA is to allow the initiated to reabsorb reality and reunite the divine lovers, awakening from the hypnotic sleep of materialism and victimization. With this aim, the Mother Mantra tradition is made up of four movements.

First movement: understanding the dream state
Second movement: taking the spirits with oneself, "the hunt for the soul"
Third movement: reuniting the divine lovers in awareness of the two in one
Fourth movement: repetition of the Mystical Marriage Mantra

Let's now see the four movements that make up the Mother Mantra practice in detail. In these movements one of the significant aspects is that of the repetition of a psychic formula. In the Mother Mantra tradition various formulas are taught, which, in truthfulness, actually work like magical formulae if used with mindfulness and knowledge. Indeed, the Mother Mantra itself is a psychic formula of the imaginal creation.

FIRST MOVEMENT

Understanding the Dream State

In the language of imaginal psychology the term *soul-making* means to develop the ability to "see" that people, things, places, and events that we perceive daily are a dream within a dream. They have no real substance; they are but shadows, mirages. Just like the moon reflected in water, they are vivid and lucid but devoid of substance. The perceptions of the objectivity of things and their materialism are deceptions that vanish into thin air like smoke the moment we wake from the dream.

Soul-making implies that we take every person, object, and event with which we come into contact back to its true imaginal nature, reminding ourselves that we are dreaming and that what we perceive are images wrought by our own dream. Soul-making thus means to take reality bit by bit and to lead it back to the soul, to the realm of Hades, to the domain of the shadows, to the depths of the eternal feminine, to the realms of the instinctual "I."

Soul-making also means to evoke the shadows that reside beyond the Great Threshold and bring them to an area where we can feasibly communicate with them: our ancestors, the archetypes, the images that inhabit the depths of our psyche, the invisible shadows that determine our thoughts and our actions.

Soul-making essentially means making everything on this side and everything beyond the Great Threshold meet at the boundary, which is beyond time and space. This boundary is a no-man's-land; it is the great Sameness and may be symbolized by androgyny. Androgyny is the symbol of the union of life and death and of all the opposites; it is the emblem of the victory of love over fear and of the meeting with the sacred, the *sacrum facere,* the capacity to self-give.

Soul-making means setting forth on the journey toward the Great Threshold, which is the land of the imaginal. The method of soul-making consists in reminding oneself, several times a day and in several ways, that you are dreaming. This is the first movement for the reabsorption of reality.

Whatever your situation may be, if you are ready to remind yourself that you are dreaming, everything around you will change instantly. If you are in a difficult situation, and you are under the impression that the events are crushing you, remember that you are the dreamer of the dream. If the surrounding reality is too hard, thick, and heavy, shout inwardly: "I am dreaming, I am dreaming, I am dreaming!" and keep on repeating this statement, which is an imaginal formula. As you repeat the formula inwardly, compare everything you see, hear, and perceive to the images of a dream.

The tantric shamans in the Himalayas have created a kind of yoga as a method for unveiling the dream state. It is called "yoga for the comprehension of the dream state" and is one of the so-called Himalayan yogas, also known as "yoga of Naropa." This yoga consists of living in awareness of the dream state. To remind oneself that one is dreaming is certainly an effective method for awakening.

SECOND MOVEMENT

Taking the Spirits with Oneself, the "Hunt for the Soul"

This is a shamanic method practiced by the shamans in Siberia and Mongolia. They understand that a person will lead a hard life until learning to take the spirits with oneself. The spirits are the most powerful expressions of a person's soul, the so-called power images. The power images are:

- ◆ The ancestors
- ◆ Places charged with a natural force, or sacred places
- ◆ Highly emotional events in one's life
- ◆ The most meaningful dreams

In this method of taking the spirits with oneself—as in the method for understanding the dream state—a psychic formula of the imaginal creation is repeated. It is simple yet extremely effective if used with awareness and knowledge. It is worthwhile remembering that experience is nothing without knowledge.

The formula for taking the spirits consists in knowing how to talk to the spirits, the gods, who are the engine of the images. It simply means saying to them, "Come with me," but in full awareness and with impeccable knowledge of what one is doing.

The Psychic Formula for the Ancestors

Thinking of your ancestors while contemplating a photograph, or when in the places they lived, or handling objects they have left, say to them, "Come with me." If you repeat this psychic formula inwardly, you will soon be pervaded by a feeling of peace, because taking your ancestors with you means appeasing their spirits.

In an imaginal vision the ancestors are powerful images projected by the psyche, and they should be thought of in a depersonalized manner—not as individuals but as dreams that the soul uses to accomplish its mission. The ancestors are not to be judged but reabsorbed, like all symbols.

The Psychic Formula for Sacred Places

Sacred places or places of power, where the natural energy is expressed in all its potential, are full of spirits to be taken with oneself. The method is to turn to the rivers, the lakes, the seas, the mountains, the plants, and the animals you come upon when you walk in the midst of nature, and say to them, "Come with me!" Taking the spirits and guardians of nature with you certainly does not mean moving them from where they are, yet it does at the same time mean taking them with you. This may seem contradictory for the mind, but it is perfectly acceptable for those who can see the complexity. That which can't be true for the mind is true for nature, which is a complex image.

Repeating the psychic formula inwardly and turning to the most powerful images of nature that can be projected by your soul, you will be pervaded by an intense feeling of joy, which is triggered by the awareness of non-duality. Even though you and the images are one single reality, which self-projects, one single soul, which self-manifests, you are nevertheless distinct: you are distinct but not separate. The principle of non-duality, also known as *advaita,* is a fundamental principle of complexity. According to this principle—even though the other is nonexistent, because everything is one—you are never alone, because everything is two in one and, considering that this state of non-duality is love, it releases pleasure and joy.

The Psychic Formula for Emotional Events

The strongest emotional events of your life—such as the emotional turmoil of your birth; the turmoil of traumatic events such as accidents, illnesses, and loss; and weddings, pregnancies, sudden intense understandings, moments of well-being, and the emotions tied to your most meaningful recurring dreams—all harbor spirits, deities, genies, demons, and demonesses of great power. Beyond good and evil, and without distinguishing the good events from the bad, fearlessly take all of these energies with you.

Repeat the psychic formula of the imaginal creation—"Come with me!"—all the while remembering the events that brought those emotions and images to you. This enables you to feel whole, complete, and allows you to relate to every part of your being, to every aspect of your soul and body, with love. It is a privilege to be true to yourself without feeling regret for the moments past and for the choices made.

The Psychic Formula for Dreams

The gods, who reside in the world of invisibility, love to visit you wearing the masks of the characters, animals, and even places of nature (mountains, rivers) or events (flying, falling) that appear in your dreams. So, dreams are privileged places for "dream-hunting." The term *dream-hunting* refers to a Siberian and Mongolian shamanic practice by which the "runaway" soul is "captured" or "restored."

For the shaman, a person who falls ill or is dealing with serious existential problems is a person who has lost his soul. Saying "he has lost his soul" rather than "he has lost fragments of soul" doesn't change the picture, because the soul is a complexity whereby everything is in the part and the part is in everything.

The method for the reabsorption of dreams entails staying a few moments in bed after waking up, recalling the images of your dreams and saying to the most meaningful images you can remember: *Come with me!*—the psychic formula of the imaginal creation.

Carrying the dream images with you throughout the day builds up a progressive process of dis-identification, distancing you from your own "I," which leads to the creation of the witnessing "I." The witnessing "I" (the Self) is an aspect of awareness capable of observing the "I" from the outside, not falling prey to its calculating mind-set bent on control or to its fears and its conditioning by categories of imposed social values. The "I" is always in a frenzy between fear and calculation, between the sense of good and bad, personal pros and cons, and doesn't understand that it is being manipulated. Its emotions are substantially fear, anguish, sadness, and solitude, because the "I" lives in the illusion of being separate from everything.

The Self is a superior trait of consciousness; it is the awareness of being distinct yet not separate from nature and the universe, partaking of the same emptiness, which is eternal instantaneity. The Self manifests with a profound sense of calm-being, an atemporal vision, a powerful energy, and a state of unfailing bliss.

THIRD MOVEMENT

Reunion of the Divine Lovers in the Awareness of the Two in One

The Self allows the reunion of the divine lovers; that is, it allows us to discover a sentiment of deep ecology, as it were. The Self sees beyond the individuals, it observes the energies that move them and, beyond objects, it observes the anima mundi.

This ability allows the reunification of light and shadow, visible and invisible; this reunion of the Father with the Mother gives way to a modification of the world's axis. With the expression *world's axis* we mean the perspective with which reality is perceived. When the Father and Mother are reunited they are both on the same plane. Death is not inferior to life; shadow is not worse than light; the invisible is not more frightening than the visible; the mystery is not to be vanquished through knowledge but understood through love. In this condition we define the world's axis as horizontal. Its horizontality symbolizes the state of nature in which no categories of power exist.

To make power possible it is necessary to make the axis vertical by introducing categories of value (true, false, good, evil, right, wrong) for governing, measuring, and predicting human nature. Then it becomes mandatory to create a metaphysical God: an entity, distinct and separate from nature, placed up high in a faraway sky, who justifies the scale of values concocted by the human mind: values that are neither supported nor justified by anything in nature. So it is for reasons of power that the two divine lovers, the two deep and fundamental aspects of the psyche, are separated: the Father is placed in a faraway sky, and the Mother sinks into the obscurantism of soulless matter or, at the best, into a sentimentally humanized naturism.

The third movement of the Mother Mantra tradition consists in reuniting the divine lovers. This is accomplished by overcoming the fear of the shadows and particularly of death. Death, meaning the end of awareness, is an illusion that exists solely in our culture; that is, in a cult that is blindly believed by the people of so-called modern society. It is a consequence of the fear that arises from having abandoned the natural state, from having betrayed nature and ruptured the universal balance for a power rush.

Death, meaning the end of awareness, doesn't exist in the animist tribes who still live in communion with nature. When the shaman beats on the drum he calls both the living and the dead to gather together. According to both the Egyptian and tantric Himalayan traditions, the end of awareness is a consequence of the fact that in death the individual feels guilty for having betrayed the pact with nature and is afraid. In fear the individual can't face the vision of what is happening. In death one's true nature is revealed: the illusion of the separate "I" ceases. In the esoteric traditions this revelation is compared to the appearance of a marvelous, brilliant, and blinding light. An individual in the grip of fear can't face this vision; with eyes closed and refusing to look, the person thus falls into the pit of unawareness and forgetfulness.

Thus the living, in dying, forgets itself. The dying will transit from death to the following birth in oblivion and will be born in oblivion. This oblivion, this forgetting, this loss of awareness is how death is experienced in our culture as a consequence of the existence of the feeling of guilt.

The fear of the shadows and the mystery of death is overcome through the repetition of a mantra called the Egyptian Mantra, which is considered the first universal variant of the Mother Mantra. In the Mother Mantra tradition the Egyptian Mantra is a privileged tool for the reunification of the divine lovers. It reunites sky and earth, light and shadow, conscious will and the will of the shadows, life and death. The Egyptian Mantra is beyond time. The tradition states that even just one repetition of this mantra paves the way inexorably, unfailingly, and impeccably to victory over fear and the illusion of death.

What follows is the exact sequence of the syllables of this extremely powerful mantra. They have never been written before or, if so, not in the correct sequence. Indeed the Egyptian Mantra has always been kept secret and has always been part of an oral tradition passed on directly from master to disciple. However it is with the consent of the visible and invisible masters that I am here revealing the correct manner to repeat the Egyptian Mantra, for the benefit of those who are able to understand the importance of soul-making and deep ecology.

⮑ The Egyptian Mantra

It is best to recite the Egyptian Mantra regularly, if even for a few minutes, once a day or a couple of times a week and anytime you feel the need for it. It should be practiced in a sitting position, with a dignified and noble posture and a straight spine. You may sit on a chair, or in the "position of the pharaoh," kneeling with haunches on heels, thighs touching, hands on your lap, palms upward, and chin toward the chest, keeping a straight back. Or you may prefer a cross-legged meditation position.

The mantra is to be said aloud, pronouncing each syllable. Every syllable of the mantra corresponds to a symbolic gesture.

1. Extend your arms in front of your body with elbows slightly bent and turn your palms toward the sky, pronouncing AKH (symbolizing a brilliant light becoming a star, the male celestial essence).

2. Turn your palms toward the earth, pronouncing BA (symbolizing the soul, the female underworld essence).

3. Turn your palms toward the sky, pronouncing KA (symbolizing the calling, the aspiration, the conscious will).

4. Turn your palms toward the earth, pronouncing SHEUT (symbolizing the instinctual will of the shadows).

5. Bring your hands together at the center of your chest, where the chakra of the heart is, pronouncing IB (symbolizing the heart, the centered being).

6. Making fists, up and in front of you with elbows slightly bent, pronounce HEKAU (symbolizing the power of the magician, one who is centered and totally in harmony with nature and the universal will; feel all your force and the power of the magician).

7. Turning your palms outward at the level of your face, pronounce SEKHEM (symbolizing your flesh and blood body, the food vehicle, the living, the sheath that bears you from birth to death).

8. Turning your palms toward yourself, pronounce SEKHU (symbolizing your body of bardo, the odor-eater, so said because it feeds on the subtle essence of things; it is the sheath that bears you from death to the following life: death and life are always simultaneous).

9. Joining your hands to cover your mouth, pronounce REN (it is the name, silence, the inspired word, the seal of secrecy).

This mantra is also very useful for bringing abundance into your life, because it connects your will and your awareness to the chthonic or subterranean residence of Hades and Persephone, the king and queen of the underworld. Hades is also known as Pluto, meaning "The Wealthy."

FOURTH MOVEMENT

The Recitation of the Mystical Marriage Mantra

This second, powerful mantra of the Mother Mantra tradition refers to the underworld bride/bridegroom. Erotic energy is considered a fundamental power, inasmuch as it is true knowledge, which is reached through inspiration and revelation. Those who repeat the Mystical Marriage Mantra refer to a spirituality of nature, a religion of freedom, and are capable of going beyond the particularities of each existing dogmatic religion, capable of spreading an effective message of peace and deep ecology. Those who recite the Mystical Marriage Mantra express a pure, free spiritual sentiment, a communion with the sacred and not with the religious social systems (the Latin word *religiosum* is distinguished from *sacrum*). If anything, the Mystical Marriage Mantra practitioner may be in resonance with the soul-making of the esoteric practitioners and the free thinkers.

A helpful context for understanding the efficacy of mantra repetition can be found in the writings of the great Indian guru Sri Aurobindo.

> The theory of the Mantra is that it is a word of power born out of the secret depths of our being where it has been brooded upon by a deeper consciousness than the mental, framed in the heart and not constructed by the intellect, held in the mind, again concentrated on by the waking mental consciousness and then thrown out silently or vocally— the silent word is perhaps held to be more potent than the spoken— precisely for the work of creation. The mantra can not only create new subjective states in ourselves, alter our physical being, reveal knowledge and faculties we did not before possess, can not only produce similar results in other minds than that of the user, but can produce vibrations in the mental and vital atmosphere which result in effects, in actions and even in the production of material forms on the physical plane.
>
> Mantra is at once a symbol, an instrument and a sound body for the divine manifestation.
>
> The function of a Mantra is to create vibrations in the inner consciousness that will prepare it for the realization of what the Mantra symbolizes and is supposed indeed to carry within itself.
>
> When one repeats a Mantra regularly, very often it begins to repeat itself within, which means that it is taken up by the inner being. In that way it is more effective.*

Sri Aurobindo on the Tantra, compiled from the writings of Sri Aurobindo by M. P. Pandit (Twin Lakes, Wisc.: Lotus Light Publications, 1999), 30.

In the tantric-shamanic Mother Mantra tradition this mantra for the mystical or alchemical marriage refers to the Name, or Nomen Arcanum. It has two variants: SAMAYA is the Nomen Arcanum of the mystical bride, and SAMAS is the Nomen Arcanum of the mystical bridegroom. Both variants are tied to the root *saman,* which is the same as in the word *shaman.* The word *shaman*—according to Mircea Eliade—probably derives from the Tungus word *saman,* which means "he who is excited," or "died and resurrected," or also "he who is in ecstasy." The Tungus *saman,* in turn, may be traced back to the Pali term *samana,* derived from the Sanskrit *sramana,* "monk."

According to the Veda, Samana is the name of the Arian god of death. For the Assyrians and Babylonians, Shamash was the god of the sun, of justice, and of divination. Saman was the sun god for the Semites of the north, and Sams was the sun god for the Semites of the south. So Saman is both the god of death and the god of life (sun). Like other deities, such as Osiris, Dionysus, Janus, and Odin, he is endowed with opposing powers and ferries the dead while accompanying the living.

The Celtic priests, the druids, celebrated the feast of Samhain—which corresponds to modern Halloween—in which the dead and the living, the light and the shadow, would meet in autumn, from October 31st to November 2nd. The feast of autumn, in agriculture, celebrates the withdrawal of the seeds into the earth, which allows them to survive the winter and bear their fruit in spring. Autumn is the dimension of death and rebirth.

In the Bhagavad Gita, Krishna says, *vedanam samavedo 'smi,* "I am the Saman of the Veda." The *Sama Veda* is one of the four canonical subsections of the Veda. The title can be translated as "The Veda of melodies," *saman* meaning "chant," "hymn," "melody," and refering to the mantras sung by the master of ceremonies of a ritual sacrifice.

According to ancient Buddhist chronicles the Buddha traveled to Mahiyangana in Sri Lanka to pay homage with one of his hairs to the god Saman, the most important divinity of the island, who is said to have welcomed him on the peak of the Sri Pada. The Sri Pada (in Singhalese Samalanakanda, the mountain of butterflies), also known as Adam's Peak, is a sacred mountain of the island of Sri Lanka. It is found in the center of the country (Ratnapura district, in the province of Sabaragamuwa) and is sacred to the god Saman.

Worshippers of the god Saman still make the pilgrimage to Sri Pada today, climbing all the way up the steep and uneven steps during the night so as to be on the peak of the mountain by dawn and witness an atmospheric marvel unique to the world: to the eyes of the observer it seems that the sun rises and sets three times. The pilgrimage to the peak of Sri Pada is accomplished by Buddhists, Hindus, Muslims, and Christians alike. On the summit (7,400 feet) is a monastery in which a very large (five and a half feet) footprint is to be found and is worshipped by the Buddhists as belonging to the Buddha. The Hindus believe it belongs to Shiva Adipadham, whereas for Christians and Muslims it is the footprint of Adam.

In tantric-shamanic yoga and in esoteric Buddhism, MAMA KO-LING SAMANTA is a mantra of great power and secrecy. *Samayà* is also a term used in esoteric Buddhism, where it may indicate a *mudra* (symbolic gesture), the enlightenment of the Buddha, and the union of the three *vajra* (skillful means) of the Buddha: word, body, and mind.

❧ The Mystical Marriage Mantra

Keeping in mind that the god Saman, who represents the divinity of nature—like the Great Mother, like Shiva as the Divine Hermaphrodite—is certainly both male and female and is androgynous in the purest and most complete sense, the two variants of the mantra to be recited are

AYA SAMAYA: for those whose visionary power imagines a female bride

AYA SAMAS: for those whose visionary power imagines a male bridegroom

The Mystical Marriage Mantra may be recited in any moment of the day, no matter what one is doing. It keeps the mind free from anxiety, bestowing more presence and lucidity. It is particularly useful in times of stress or danger, because it offers the protection of the invisible lover.

ᴄ The Silent Practice of the Mystical Marriage Mantra
It is particularly advisable to recite the Mystical Marriage Mantra in the evening in bed, on the verge of sleep, so as to entrust your slumber to the embrace of the underworld bride/bridegroom. The invisible lover accompanies you in every transit: from life to death and from death to life, from waking to sleeping (which is a little death) and from sleeping to waking. In fact you transit in every single moment of life: at the end of every breath, before the next breath starts, every time a thought finishes, before the next thought surfaces. The invisible lover is always with you, embracing you, whispering in your ears the loving warning: "Don't be afraid."

Repeat the Mystical Marriage Mantra before falling asleep, for a few minutes or even for just a few seconds, to confirm your alliance with the invisible soul. You may wake up during the night and hear that the mantra is repeating itself, by itself, inside. The mantra is able to trigger a kind of "automatic power," whereby it repeats by itself. Indeed, as mentioned earlier, the Mother Mantra is also defined as "the automatic means."

ᴄ The Vocal Repetition of the Mystical Marriage Mantra
Your state of awareness and psychophysical energy levels are enhanced nearly immediately through the vocal recitation of the mantra. The breathing should be deep, slow, and complete.

Recite AYA during exhalation, and SAMAYA or SAMAS during inhalation. It isn't easy to produce a sound while inhaling—in this case SAMAYA or SAMAS. A kind of in-sucking sound should be made. All the air should be expelled during the exhalation with AYA, gently contracting the abdomen toward the end. The quality of breathing is conditioned by the exhalation, so if you breathe out well and fully, then you will breathe in well too.

To achieve the immediate enhancement of the state of awareness and psychophysical energy levels, eleven consecutive, complete deep vocal repetitions will suffice.

With sixty or more repetitions you will achieve enhancement of the state of consciousness and the opening of the energetic meridians and chakra—the psychophysical energy centers in the subtle physiology of yoga—to cosmic energy and inspiration. Ideas—which are eidola, which are the gods—flow freely through the doors of the chakras when they have been opened.

It is important to remember to always pronounce AYA while exhaling and SAMAS or SAMAYA while inhaling. As the great tantric yogi Abhinavagupta says: "In exhalation is the day, in inhalation is the night."* Inhalation means bringing in the spirit; exhalation means letting it out. When we exhale we project reality, we manifest, we give witness to everything we see, hear, or perceive. The spirit is light, and to expand it outside ourselves means to illuminate, to manifest, to give witness; to inhale is to reabsorb reality, to withdraw projections. For "soul-making," the Name or Nomen Arcanum is always to be inhaled, never exhaled. If you wish to restore every thing, person, event, and place to its true nature, which is image, projection, then it must be reabsorbed knowingly. To inhale the Numen Arcanum allows this knowing reabsorption; it allows us to dematerialize reality and restore our relationship with invisibility. This means to reestablish the primeval balance, the universal order, between light and shadow, death and life, dreaming and waking, and all of the other opposites that have been broken by today's civilization, known for its fear and ignorance of the invisible worlds.

---

*Abhinavagupta, *Tantraloka, Luce del Tantra.*

5

The Spiritual Practices
of the Morning
and Evening

THE MORNING AND
EVENING STAR EXERCISES

These two practices are simple but extremely effective. They are only a taste of the vast and articulate amount of spiritual exercises and healing rituals that make up the Mother Mantra tradition. Nevertheless, the heart of the Mother Mantra experience is contained in these simple exercises, and their constant and regular practice will open the chakras and energy meridians, thus enabling ideas and feelings of utmost joy and elevation to reach you, allowing you to lead a serene and inspired life.

ʔ The Morning and Evening Star

The main aim of these spiritual exercises is to enable the contact with ideas—that is, gods—of a creative and lovable kind. Practice the Evening Star in the evening and the Morning Star every morning, even if only for a few minutes, before sleeping and after waking. In both practices you may repeat the Mystical Marriage Mantra inwardly, breathing through your nostrils, or aloud, breathing through your mouth. A slow, calm breath is advisable for the evening practice, whereas a deep and energetic breath is preferable for the morning practice. Both exercises may be done either standing or lying down. Both Stars may be done in a sitting position (seated on a chair, back straight, feet on the floor, hands in lap with palms upward), in a meditative posture, or in the pharaoh position. The important thing is to maintain a noble and dignified posture. And remember, you should chant AYA SAMAYA if your visionary power imagines a female bride and AYA SAMAS if you visionary power imagines a male bridegroom.

✑ The Evening Star

Through the Evening Star practice, known as the "withdrawal of projections," you will become accustomed to treating reality as a figment of your imagination, a dream. The more you practice the less you will consider yourself the victim of events and the more you will become their friend, partner, lover. It helps you to become acquainted with the substantial impermanence of every apparition, to sever the attachments that cause suffering; it also helps to widen your outlook and sleep well, profoundly. Night after night, fear vanishes.

1. Lie in bed on your back with your eyes closed. Open both arms and legs to a six-pointed star position. The points of the star are the hands, the feet, the head, and the groin.

2. Imagine there is an opening in the middle of your chest corresponding to the heart chakra, and inhale through it. While you inhale, repeat the mantra SAMAS or SAMAYA and imagine you are absorbing energy in the form of light through the heart chakra. The energy spreads throughout your body and is returned to the universe through the six points of the star. While you exhale, repeat AYA.

3. While breathing in, imagine that you are reabsorbing into your heart chakra all the images, or projections, of your day; that is, everything you

have seen, heard, or experienced, seeing it as a dream, an illusion.

4. While breathing out, those images go back to being organs, body, soul; they then leave the body through the six points of the star, and vanish.

ᖇ The Morning Star

The Morning Star practice, known as the "reawakening of the energies able to influence the imaginal creation," harmonizes you with the universal forces, unburdening you of the weight of the cage of the "I," which makes you feel separate and isolated from the rest of the universe. This allows you to accomplish inspired, compassionate actions, giving joy to yourself and those with whom you may come into contact throughout your day.

1. Stand with both arms and legs slightly open.
2. Inhale light through the six points of your star reciting, the mantra SAMAS or SAMAYA.
3. Exhale light through the chakra of the heart, reciting the mantra AYA. Keep your eyes half closed, pointing to the infinite, beyond what you can see.
4. Dissolve your "I" in the light that circulates powerfully through your whole being.

With the Evening Star reality is reabsorbed, projections are withdrawn and the world is re-conducted to its true nature, which is imaginal creation. With the Morning Star you reawaken the energies, which enable you to act upon the imaginal creation. If necessary the spiritual exercises may also be done during the day to dissolve tormenting apparitions or to charge your energy for an important event.

Consistent practice allows the deep subconscious to assimilate the ability to withdraw projections and to reawaken the energies to act on the imaginal creation, further allowing a radical shift in the way that reality is perceived and related to. If you have very little time, just give them a few precious seconds, but try to do so regularly. You will see your life change for the better, guided by your most unperturbed and farsighted ideas.

THE PRACTICE OF REMEMBRANCE

The Practice of Remembrance is accomplished through the repetition of promises, promises that keep the remembrance of the spirit of the Mother Mantra alive. These promises, which guide the actions of the Guardians of the Mother Mantra tradition, will also help you along your path if you join them to a regular practice of the Morning and Evening Star.

The promises should be recited in the midst of nature, whispered to the trees, to the earth, and to the sky, with both hands clasped to the chakra of the heart.

AYA SAMAS/SAMAYA, I promise to remember that I am loved. AYA SAMAS/SAMAYA.

AYA SAMAS/SAMAYA, I promise to love abundantly. AYA SAMAS/ SAMAYA.

AYA SAMAS/SAMAYA, I promise to not put off my awakening. AYA SAMAS/SAMAYA.

AYA SAMAS/SAMAYA, I promise to cultivate beauty, in contact with nature. AYA SAMAS/SAMAYA.

AYA SAMAS/SAMAYA, I promise to practice the spiritual exercise of the morning and evening. AYA SAMAS/SAMAYA.

AYA SAMAS/SAMAYA, I promise to follow a healthy diet. AYA SAMAS/SAMAYA.

AYA SAMAS/SAMAYA, I promise to cultivate the fire of dumo. AYA SAMAS/SAMAYA.

The Practice of Remembrance, together with the practice of the Morning Star and the Evening Star, will make you a Carrier of the Mother Mantra. Always remember who you are and face events with a positive attitude, because nothing can vanquish you if not your own distraction or forgetfulness. Remember who you are!

THE FIVE SPIRITUAL RITUALS OF THE MORNING AND THE EVENING

The five spiritual morning and evening rituals were passed on to me directly by my teacher of yoga and shamanism, Michael Williams. He declared that of all the things he had learned, nothing was more powerful and effective than these spiritual exercises.

More than thirty years after the day that he revealed them to me on the beach of Weligama, I can confirm that in their very simplicity they express all the deepest secrets of yoga and shamanism. I have spent the past thirty years traveling and researching the many differing traditions for reaching longevity, realization, and liberation. I have known many peoples, cultures, and secrets. I have witnessed shamanic rituals and ceremonies of many a kind, from Mongolia to Siberia, from South America to Tibet, but my experience is that his clams for the effectiveness of these rituals is valid. They are the key to a long, healthy, happy, and inspired life.

The morning and evening spiritual exercises from the Mother Mantra tradition are, par excellence, the sacred rituals that reestablish the primeval order, the universal balance; they reconcile the human and the Divine in a partnership that brings divinity back into nature and reunite the Father with the Mother. The erotic union of all the opposites turns a person into an inspired means, a vehicle of pleasure and creativity.

If you wish to live a happy and inspired life then the spiritual exercises of the morning and the evening are the method. Furthermore, they really are the secret for staying young. Aging, meaning a sclerotizing mind and a shriveling, hardened body, is not actually a natural process. I have understood that in natural aging the body becomes subtle and supple, not thick and rigid. It is only fear that makes people thicken up and grow hardened.

The secret of success and well-being lies in our endocrine glands, nerve plexuses, and spinal ganglions, which correspond to the chakras in the subtle body. The art of the spiritual morning and evening exercises is ancient and is founded on the knowledge of the chakras, of their way of working, of how they tune in to melodies, energies, and cosmic laws.

The Melting of Fear

The morning and evening rituals melt fear at a very profound level, tapping in to the neuro-vegetative system, leaving a sense of marvel and gratitude in its stead. True old age brings further reasons for feeling grateful, as it is a reunion with the whole and culminates in an apotheosis of awareness, which is love and not the end or death, as it is called; it means giving oneself, not losing oneself.

These spiritual exercises are so simple that anyone can do them! I hope you may practice them for the benefit of all beings, and that you may also pass them on, so that love might vanquish death and fear be overcome and dispelled. These rituals, passed on through the Mother Mantra tradition, were among the first that Michael taught me, and I shall describe them exactly as he did to me.

The Five Elements

Each of the five spiritual exercises is based on one of the five elements of Indian philosophy: *akasha* (space), *tejas* (fire), *vayu* (air), *prithvi* (earth), and *jala* (water). These five elements are understood to be the basic constituents of nature.

In each of the five rituals the physical and the psychic are brought together. The physical gestures that are done before the psychic gestures in the rituals are movements that act on the chakras and on the *nadi;* that is, on the system of subtle energies that govern our body and our life. For example, the psychic gesture of full acceptance of this world and this life, accomplished in the Akasha ritual given below, will trigger a feeling of self-faith, which works as a powerful antidepressant and motivating factor. Once a given series of physical and psychic gestures is performed they remain in one's memory and gradually release the desired effects over time, increasing in intensity the more frequently the ritual is accomplished, as its memory sinks into the automatisms of the psyche.

The Son and the Mother

Each of the five exercises below are broken in to two parts: a Son experience and a Mother experience. All things come into being, into reality, from an act of intuition, from primordial images—the Mother experience. Thus the energy becomes matter or substance expressed in our world—the Son experience. The Son represents the energetic-corporeal experience, while the Mother represents the visionary experience. Because in our day and age we are much more familiar with the corporal dimension rather than with the visionary, it is customary for a corporeal, sensory experience to precede a visionary one. Hence my decision to present the Son experience before the Mother experience.

⸙ Akasha, Space—The Spiritual Rite of Reconciliation

In the vision of non-duality the element space is itself the reconciler, because subject and object are illusions. When two individuals get in touch, there is not a meeting and then a separation; they are always already qualities of space, unified. What we can really experience in the ritual is just the pure essence of dynamic space.

↶ Son Experience—Energy-Body Experience, Exploration of Space

1. Standing position. Open arms at shoulder height, palms downward. Deeply inhale through nostrils (fig. 5.1, step 1).
2. Exhaling through nose, turn torso left, placing right palm on left shoulder and left hand on right flank. Rest chin on back of right hand and turn torso as far left as you can, feeling the torsion (fig. 5.1, step 2).
3. Inhaling, turn to the front and extend the arms (fig. 5.1, step 3).
4. Exhaling, turn torso right. Rest left palm on right shoulder and right

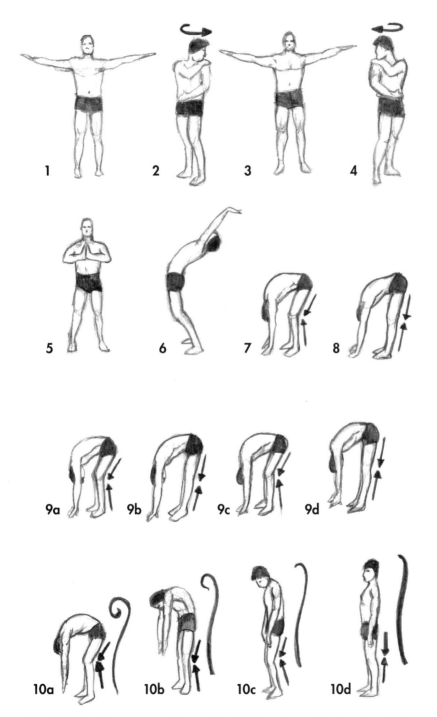

Fig. 5.1. Son Experience—Energy-Body Experience, Exploration of Space

hand on left flank. Rest chin on back of left hand and turn torso as far right as possible (fig. 5.1, step 4).

5. Inhaling, turn to the front and join palms in prayer in front of chest. Exhale here (fig. 5.1, step 5).

6. Inhaling, raise both arms up and back, arching the spine backward (fig. 5.1, step 6).

7. Exhaling, bring your hands to the floor in front of your feet, knees slightly bent. Let your head relax completely downward (fig. 5.1, step 7).

8. Inhaling, try to extend your knees as far as you can without lifting your hands from the floor (fig. 5.1, step 8).

9. Repeat steps 7 and 8 two more times (fig. 5.1, step 9 a–d).

10. Inhaling slowly and deeply, straighten up, taking care to keep knees slightly bent until your spine is in a perfect upright position (fig. 5.1, step 10 a–d).

～ Mother Experience—Visionary Experience, Exploration of Time

To do this practice you need to visualize the *bindu* chakra, a small growth of the brain at the top of the head. In the old days the Hindu priests of the brahmin caste used to make a ponytail at that point to help them maintain their perception of the bindu chakra. This chakra secretes drops of very precious liquid called *amrita,* the nectar of the gods. This secretion is produced if the chakra is stimulated, or spontaneously in certain "passages" in life, such as the shift from adolescence to adulthood, or from maturity to senior age.

1. Sit in a position for meditation. For at least three minutes, breathing deeply through the mouth, whisper the Mystical Marriage Mantra (AYA during exhalation, and SAMAYA or SAMAS during inhalation) (fig. 5.2, step 1).

2. With your hands over your heart, visualize all the possible worlds you can (various epochs, eras, places, etc.). Realize that the choice of this world is determined by a necessity of the soul.

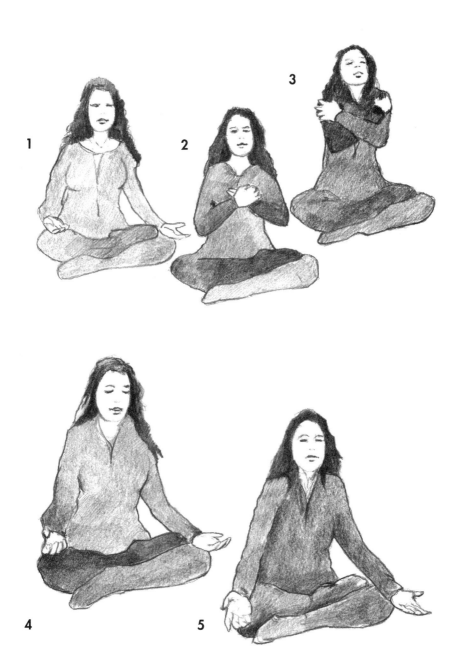

Fig. 5.2. Mother Experience—
Visionary Experience, Exploration of Time

With your hands on your heart, visualize all the lives you might have had (if, for example, you had married one man instead of another, or had studied something else, or accepted another job that day . . .). Realize that the choice of this life is determined by an intrinsic need of the soul, even if it may be beyond the mind's understanding (fig. 5.2, step 2).

3. Make the sign of triple acceptance of this world and this life. It is the sign of supreme re-pacification: left hand on right shoulder, right hand on left shoulder, head, eyes, and tongue turned upward. The gesture expresses the firm intention to taste the nectar of this world and this life. To do so correctly, turn your head up and slightly back, curl the tip of your tongue up and back to touch on the soft palate as far back as you can, and roll your eyeballs up under closed eyelids. Push with your tongue and eyeballs so as to perceive a white light behind your eyelids (fig. 5.2, step 3).

4. Bring your head to its normal position, eyes (still closed) to the front and to the infinite, relax the tongue, and feel the amrita descending from the bindu chakra to the whole body, experiencing the bliss (fig.5.2, step 4).

5. Put your hands on your lap with elbows extended and palms up in front of your knees. Touch the earth in front of your knees with the tips of your middle fingers if you are seated on the ground, otherwise open your hands wide. Pray that the amrita might multiply and nourish all the creatures in the nine empty universes.* In exchange ask to receive inspired visions (fig. 5.2, step 5).

6. Last but not least, with hands on heart, recite the "Vow of Faithfulness to Oneself" with the following psychic formula of the imaginal creation: *In the dance of space-time, I am the calling of my soul.* Seal the psychic formula with a whispered recitation of the Mystical Marriage Mantra (see page 71).

---

*Nine is a magic, esoteric number in the Mother Mantra tradition, and "empty" represents the belief that emptiness is the real substance of everything—*reality*, the Mother Mantra tells us, is essentially *void*.

ॐ Tejas, Fire—The Spiritual Ritual of Love

Here we ignite the fire element qualities of passion and love.

∾ Son Experience—Body-Energy Experience, Lighting the Flame

1. Kneel with haunches on heels or, if you can, backside on the floor with your feet on the outside of your buttocks (fig. 5.3, step 1). You can put a cushion under your backside for comfort. Keep your hands in the praying position in front of your chest (fig. 5.3, step 2). This is called the "Flame Position" and helps to stretch the anterior thigh muscles and relax the leg and pelvis joints.

2. Keep this posture for the Mother Experience.

∾ Mother Experience—Visionary Experience, Kindling the Flame

Phase One

Duration: one or two minutes.

3. Place your hands on your lap, thumb tips touching each other. Keep silent, listening to your heartbeat and the pauses of silence. Inwardly repeat the following formula of the imaginal creation: *This body is a magical apparition, a dream, a mirage; it is like a flash of lightning, appearing and vanishing, appearing and vanishing, like a wave in emptiness.* Keep your eyes half-open, looking in front of you without focusing on anything (fig. 5.3, step 3).

Phase Two

Duration: a couple of minutes.

4. Open your arms in an all-embracing gesture. The hands—palms up—should be relaxed. Start breathing mainly with your chest, inhalation slightly longer than exhalation. Breathe through a slightly open mouth (fig. 5.3, step 4).

5. While exhaling, bend your torso slightly forward, as though your body wanted to take flight, reciting the mantra AYA (fig. 5.3, step 5).

6. While inhaling, bring your torso back to the erect, relaxed position, reciting the name of your underworld bridegroom or bride, SAMAS or SAMAYA (fig.5.3, step 6).

Phase Three

Duration: one minute.

7. With your hands on your lap, repeat the words *love* and *harmony* silently (fig. 5.3, step 7).

Phase Four

Duration: a couple of minutes.

8 and 9. Repeat the all-embracing gesture from phase two, whereby you embrace the invisibility that surrounds and wraps you, repeating the Mystical Marriage Mantra as you bend forward (fig. 5.3, steps 8 and 9). Repeat this movement six times, mentally reciting one of the following six phrases each time you bend forward.

I am grateful for my dreams.

I am grateful for everything that could have been, yet wasn't.

I am grateful for everything that was in this life that I don't remember (my life in the womb, my birth, my childhood, my adolescence, my adulthood).

I am grateful for my ancestors.

I am grateful for what I don't remember from past lives.

I am grateful for my body of bardo.

Phase Five

Duration: one or two minutes.

10. Return to the upright position with your hands in your lap (fig. 5.3, step 10). Stay silent and listen to your heart beat and to the pauses of silence between the beats. Now you are in Sameness, and you can simultaneously "see" all that is living and all that is dying.

This practice yields love for your fellows and devotion for an idea or ideal. It also helps to heal problems of a sentimental kind.

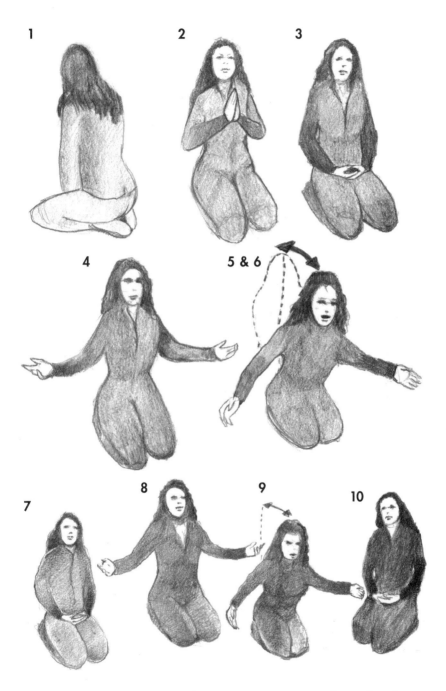

Fig. 5.3. Son Experience—Body-Energy Experience, Lighting the Flame; and Mother Experience—Visionary Experience, Kindling the Flame

❧ *Vayu, Air—The Ritual of Nonexistence*

In these exercises we will tap in to the power the air element has to dissolve the body's walls and bring us into the dimension of nonexistence.

➤ Son Experience—Body-Energy Experience, the Rising of the Snake

1. Sit on your heels and lean your forehead on the floor, keeping your haunches on your heels (fig. 5.4, step 1).

2. During a long and deep inhalation, lift up your backside, slightly rolling your head forward so that the point of contact with the floor shifts from your forehead toward the top of your head, stretching the neck pleasantly and pushing the chin toward the chest, thus stimulating the fifth chakra in the subtle body, which corresponds to the pharyngeal plexus, the inside of the neck, and the thyroid gland in the physical body (fig. 5.4, step 2).

3. Stay in this position for a moment with full lungs, contracting the anal sphincter and the pelvic floor (*mula bandha*). This will give a powerful upward thrust to the *kundalini* energy: all the latent psychophysical energy in the human being, which is depicted as a sleeping snake in two and a half coils at the base of the spine. This practice awakens kundalini and pushes it up the spinal column, making the energy available for several vital, emotional, mental, and spiritual functions.

4. Exhaling, relax the pelvic floor and bring the haunches back to the heels, slowly bringing your forehead back in contact with the floor.

5. Repeat the practice for three minutes consecutively.

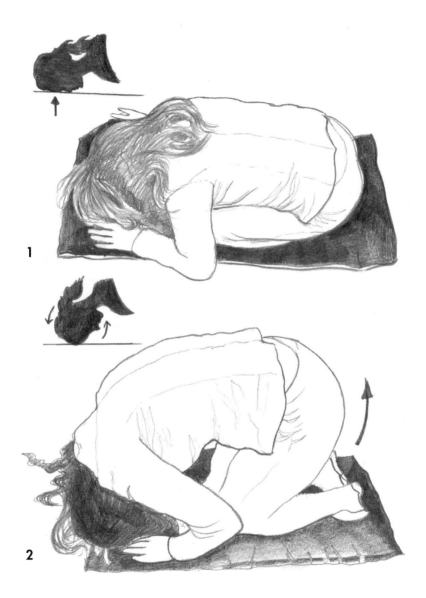

Fig. 5.4. Son Experience—Body-Energy Experience,
the Rising of the Snake

ᕀ Mother Experience—Visionary Experience, the Flight in the Wind

1. Sit in a position for meditation near an open door or window or find a quiet place outside in the open air (fig. 5.5). If it is winter cover up well but be sure to leave your face, hands, forearms, feet, and shins naked.

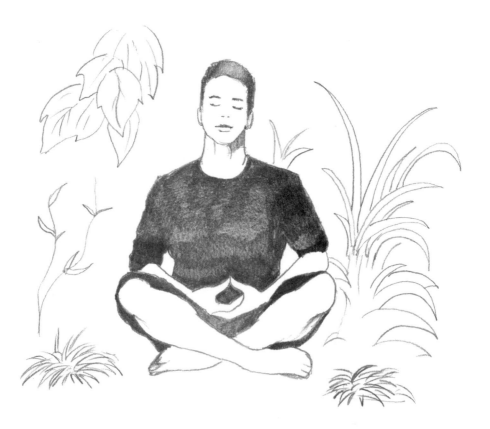

Fig. 5.5. Mother Experience—Visionary Experience,
the Flight in the Wind

2. While meditating, feel the outside air as it touches the inside of your body. With this touching and separating—incessant touching and separating—of the inside and outside air, the limits of your bodily "I" seem to vanish. Gradually you feel that the outside air is coming from places farther and farther away and the inside air from deeper and more intimate places.

3. When it seems that your bodily "I" has been utterly dissolved in the dance of vayu, the wind, stay still for a few more moments, reciting the Mystical Marriage Mantra with deep, heartfelt gratitude.

ᕽ *Prithvi, Earth—The Spiritual Homage to the Ancestors*

The Earth is our ethnic, familial, and cultural background. It is the element that represent our roots and these exercises allow us to uncover those roots.

ᕽ Son Experience—Energy-Body Experience, Arrow and Mountain

1. Standing, join hands in prayer in front of the chest (fig. 5.6, step 1).

2. Inhale while arching back the spine and lifting your hands upward (fig. 5.6, step 2).

3. Exhaling, bow forward, clutching your legs with your arms and pulling the body toward your thighs. Keep your legs as straight as you can and bring your forehead as close as you can to your legs (fig. 5.6, step 3).

4. Inhaling, place your hands on the floor beside your feet (fig. 5.6, step 4).

5. Thrust your left leg backward, place your left knee and foot on the floor (fig. 5.6, step 5).

6. Arch your spine and head backward, thus stretching the abdomen and the left thigh muscles (fig. 5.6, step 6).

7. Exhaling, thrust your right leg back and place it next to the left. If possible, flatten both feet on the floor and push both heels down. Look toward your belly button (fig. 5.6, step 7). (This is the position of the mountain.)

8. Inhaling, bring your left foot forward between your hands, placing your right knee on the floor and arching your spine and head backward, stretching the abdomen and right thigh muscles (position of the right arrow) (fig. 5.6, step 8).

9. Exhaling, bring your right foot forward, level with the left one. Clutch your legs again and pull your body toward the thighs. Keep your legs as straight as you can and bring your forehead as close as possible to your legs (fig. 5.6, step 9).

10. Inhaling, come up to a standing position and arch backward, raising your arms (fig. 5.6, step 10).

11. Come back to a straight spine and join your hands in prayer in front of your chest (fig. 5.6, step 11).

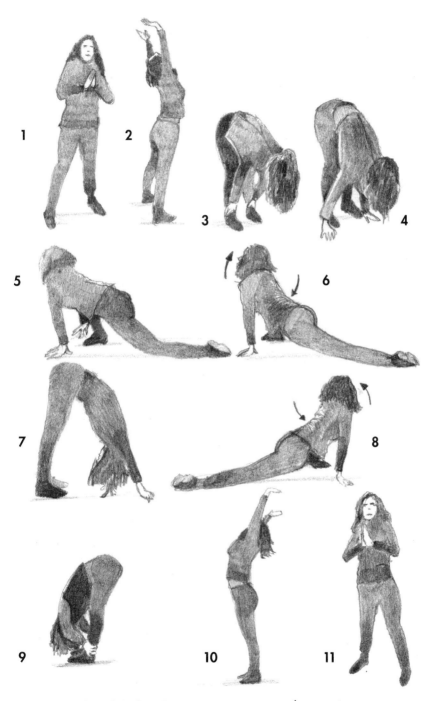

Fig. 5.6. Son Experience—Energy-Body Experience,
Arrow and Mountain

ᖋ Mother Experience—Visionary Experience, the Background

1. Sit on your heels with your hands on your lap (right hand over left), thumbs touching. Visualize that you are in front of an ancestor to whom you wish to show reverence. Repeat the Mother Mantra nine times (fig. 5.7, step 1 a–b).

2. Bring your hands to the prayer position in front of your chest and breathe normally, allowing the impressions of this revered ancestor to surface freely in your mind (fig. 5.7, step 2).

3. Open your arms and then clap twice briskly, making a short, sharp sound to send away any negative surrounding presence coming from the past (fig. 5.7, step 3 a–b).

4. Inhaling deeply, slide your hands down your thighs and onto the floor in front of your knees, joining the thumbs and index fingers to make a triangle. Rest your head on this triangle (fig. 5.7, step 4 a–c). Stay in this position for a few normal breaths, expressing your devotion and reverence.

5. Then, inhaling deeply and sliding your hands up your thighs, come back to a seated position with hands in prayer position (fig. 5.7, step 5). Take a deep breath as you recite SAMAS or SAMAYA, and breathe out with AYA.

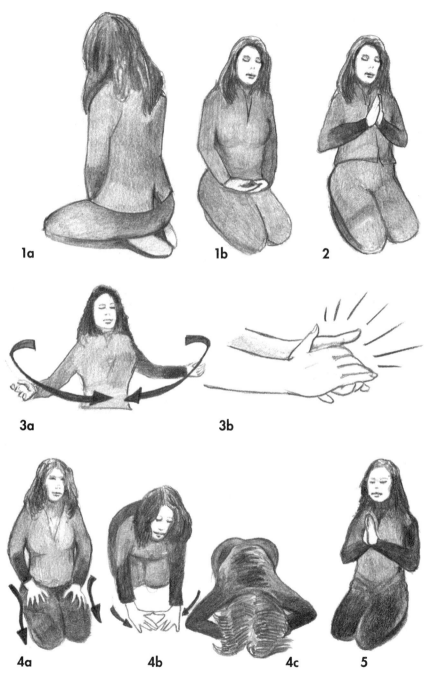

Fig. 5.7. Mother Experience—Visionary Experience,
the Background

ॐ Jala, Water—The Sword of Light

Water is the element of original purity of all things. Everything is pure at the beginning; the Sword of Light is a tool of repurification.

∾ Son Experience—Energy-Body Experience, the Triangle and the Ball

1. Lie on your back. Lift your legs straight up so they are perpendicular to the floor. Keep your toes pointed toward your face. Whisper the Mystical Marriage Mantra nine times with deep circular breathing through the mouth. The body shapes a triangle (fig. 5.8, step 1).

2. Bend your knees toward the torso (fig. 5.8, step 2).

3. Open your arms at shoulder height, placing the palms on the floor. Exhaling with AYA, let both knees fall to the right while your face twists to the left. Imagine that you are a spinning ball (fig. 5.8, step 3).

4. Inhaling with SAMAS or SAMAYA, bring your bent knees back to the chest and head and arms back to center (fig. 5.8, step 4).

5. Exhaling with AYA, let your knees fall to the left, while your face twists to the right. Keep on imagining that you are a spinning ball (fig. 5.8, step 5).

6. Inhaling with SAMAS or SAMAYA, bring your knees back to your chest and head and arms back to center.

7. Straighten your legs upward (fig. 5.8, step 6).

8. Repeat at least three times.

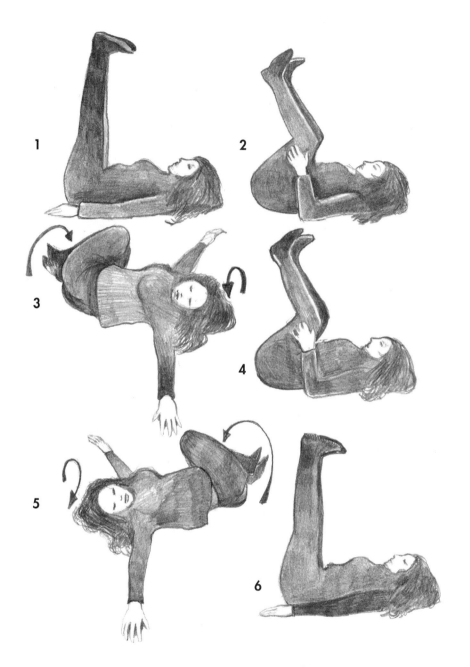

Fig. 5.8. Son Experience—Energy-Body Experience,
the Triangle and the Ball

∾ Mother Experience—Visionary Experience, the Sword of Light

1. Begin in a standing position. Open your arms, right arm straight up, left arm straight down while inhaling deeply with SAMAS or SAMAYA. Imagine that you are holding all the negativity of the world in your arms (fig. 5.9, step 1).

2. Exhaling, recite AYA and bring your hands toward each other as though you were catching a sphere (fig. 5.9, step 2). Imagine that you are holding a globe of light in your hands, in which you pour all the negativity caught by the movement of your arms, and see it transform into light. Smile.

3. Open your arms, inhaling and repeating SAMAS or SAMAYA, this time stretching the left arm up and the right arm down (fig. 5.9, step 3).

4. Exhaling with AYA, bring your hands to catch the sphere and absorb the negativity into the globe of light as before (fig. 5.9, step 4). Smile.

5. Repeat the gathering of light three times to each side then bring your arms to your sides.

6. Lift one arm straight in front of you, pointing your index and middle fingers, folding the others. Imagine the arm and two straight fingers are a sword of light (fig. 5.9, step 5).

7. Bring the sword of light down firmly, bending your knees and saying the mantra HEKA (fig. 5.9, step 6). You may remember that the word HEKAU from the Egyptian Mantra means "magician." HEKA is the "magic" that dissolves all negativity. When you lower the sword and pronounce the mantra HEKA, you feel that you can cut through darkness and shatter obstacles.

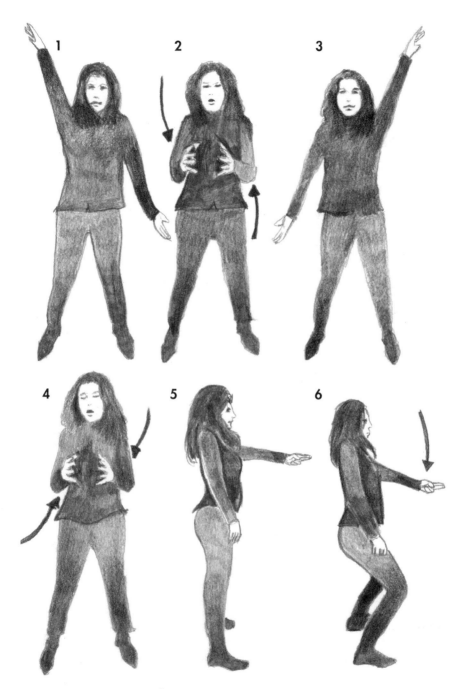

Fig. 5.9. Mother Experience—Visionary Experience,
the Sword of Light

⌇ Rest in the Light

Sit on the floor with your knees bent toward your chest. Clasp your knees with your arms and rest your head on your knees, keeping them as close as you can to your body. Stay in this rest position, which gently stretches your spine, for a few moments.

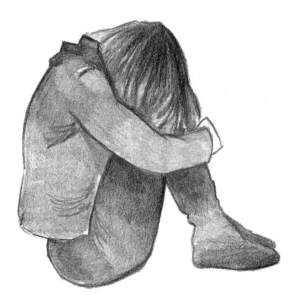

Fig. 5.10. Rest position

⌇

The great thing about the spiritual morning and evening rituals is that they take very little time and don't need to be repeated for very long, but they do have to be done regularly. The ideal moment for doing these exercises is in the morning before you start your day and in the evening just before going to bed. Ideally the first three should be done in the morning and the remaining two in the evening.

Within a few days of regular practice the benefits will be obvious and will encourage you to carry on. After just a month you will notice that you are healthier and in a better general mood. After three to six months you will notice without a doubt that your mind is lucid and inspired. Over the years your body will stay young, thanks to the chakras working properly. People will ask you for advice, convinced that you harbor some kind of magical secret. The truth is always more simple than the mind expects. The five spiritual morning and evening exercises from the Mother Mantra tradition are an amazing example of efficient simplicity.

Thanks to the activation of the deep circular breathing cycles, along with the repetition of the Mystical Marriage Mantra, the body quickly reacquires its ability to breathe freely. This ability will be performed by the body whenever deemed necessary, night or day, thus maintaining an optimal energy level and triggering a natural toxin eliminating process.

The mental attitude of the practitioner is fundamental. Practice as though you are performing a magic ritual, because that is precisely what you are doing. Performing these exercises as simple gymnastics will defeat their function and use. They are prayers that allow humanity and divinity to communicate through the wonderful energy portals called chakras. When performing the rituals I suggest that you create a sacred time-space in which you are sure not to be disturbed. You may like to listen to music, preferably relaxing and soft, and it's always a good idea to light a candle and some incense as an offering of light and fragrance for the spirits.

6

Rite, Myth, and Compassion

THE SEVEN MESSENGERS

The soul has seven great messengers: pain, illness, old age, death, sleep, sexual passion, and research, all of which are objects of study in all the sacred traditions.

To understand pain is to free oneself from suffering. To understand illness means to loosen any state of unease, disturbance, or malaise. To understand old age means to vanquish aging. To understand death means to sever death at its roots. To understand sleep means to nourish the magic of the so-called waking state, which is also, in truth, a dream state. To understand sexuality means to include the genital experience in the state of immovable pleasure, pleasure that is unceasing because it does not depend on any external object. To understand research means to already be on a path.

To understand the seven messengers means to heed the soul's calling. The soul beckons from the invisible realms, from the lunar worlds of shadow, from the dwelling of Hades. Its voices are the great offspring of death, the call of the ability to self-give, to create beyond oneself.

The soul is the invisible part of everything; it calls us back to the mystery, to the sacred, to the sacrum facere, to the rite, to creativity, with the awareness that every creation brings with it a death. The true rite is always a ritual of sacrifice, whereby our "I" gives back control and power to nature and plunges into the immensity of beauty.

If Minos had returned the white bull, symbol of power, to Poseidon, he would not have had to face the consequences of refusing to sacrifice it: the rage of Poseidon that was unleashed on him, Theseus, and all their offspring.

The gods are the body organs, and they harbor anger until the sacrificial rite is accomplished, until the "I" sacrifices its own illusion of having power, of maintaining control over nature and body. The sacrifice reestablishes the universal balance, the primeval order, which was destroyed by the betrayal of the pact with nature.

Mental knowledge, separated from the body's feeling and from love, isolates a human being from the rest of the universe. Consequently, the seven messengers—such as illness, pain, sex—are a great resource for us. They are indeed our greatest patrimony, the chance to turn back and to understand that something has been left unaccomplished. They are the soul's beckoning to not forget the shadow from whence we come and to where we are directed. This shadow is not evil at all; on the contrary, it is our true nature in the emptiness, emptiness itself. It is not nothing; it is the clear light of emptiness. This shadow is the pure light of the primary essence, free from any deception, from any mirage, blunder, or illusion. Thus it is the light that enlightens; that is, the light whereby it is possible to understand the true nature of everything. Those who have caught a glimpse of this light even once in their lifetime are said to be enlightened, because light is clear understanding and full awareness.

To see the light, darkness is necessary. The seven messengers summon you to undertake the journey into the night, beyond the Great Threshold, into the realms of Hades, into the worlds of invisibility, into the dimension of the soul. The orgasm is a little death (la petite mort) in which the logical thought sequence is shattered and the temporal sequence of events is atomized. Sleep is a little death during which one descends to and returns from the underworld. Illness and states of suffering are also little deaths.

Only old age and the great death have no apparent return. In actual fact there is no return because there is no journey, inasmuch as the journey is an unveiling and seeing of that which has always been. This journey is a path along which there is no movement. It is the "journey of the hero," made up of moments that are one within the other, in a hologram of emotions and beauty. These moments are the calling; the hesitation when faced with the calling; the approach to the Great Threshold; the encounter with the guardians of the threshold, Scylla and Charybdis, who represent the common sense of good and evil and the discrimination of the opposites; the victory over the guardians and the crossing of the Great Threshold; the great trial of initiation; the conquest of the magic sword; the purification rite that allows the hero to return to No Man's Land; and the return (for further reading, see Joseph Campbell's *The Hero with a Thousand Faces*).

When the answer to the calling is "No," the suffering is useless and to no avail. When the answer to the calling is "Yes," then the seven messengers, the great demons, reveal their true nature and show themselves to be our most loving protectors. They are actually the seven fundamental aspects of our underworld bride/bridegroom, and they manifest as the great psychopomps—Hecate, Hermes—who ferry us to the chthonic realms. They are the direct emanations of Hades and Persephone, the king and queen of the underworld.

Saying "Yes" to the mystical marriage reestablishes the universal order, the harmony between human and nature, between will and awareness. We suffer because our awareness is separate from the true willpower that makes events happen. The latter is indeed profoundly instinctive and animist; it is shadow.

RITE AND THERAPY

A desacralized therapy is born from the "I," and its aim is to strengthen the structure of the "I" and cannot do this without considering the body as a material object. A therapy that is induced from the outside, based on categories of power in technical-scientific knowledge, builds up a relationship of power between a therapist, who expects to know, and a patient, who expects not to know. This relationship is based on the law of cause and effect, animated by evidence, contrary to what science should lead us to think. Quantum mechanics states, indeed, that what we see is not what is.

Quantum physics shows us that at a subatomic level, matter is a wave that spreads in emptiness and behaves as a particle only when observed. It is not possible to calculate both the speed and the position of a quantum particle simultaneously, because the more accurate the calculus on its position is, the less accurate the calculus on its speed is, and vice versa. This property, known as Heisenberg's principle of indeterminacy, does not depend on the limits of our instrumentation but rather on the intrinsic traits of matter itself. Subatomic particles appear out of nowhere for infinitesimal fractions of a second and then vanish again without a trace. They are waves that behave as particles when they are observed.

This was already well known in ancient times: the dancing Shiva described in the ancient Vedic Hindu texts is depicted as the soul itself of the big bang and of the dance of matter in emptiness. Chidambaram, the center of the universe where the dance takes place, is in our hearts. Let's see what the great Indologist, Coomaraswamy, has to say about it:

> In the night of Brahma, nature is inert and cannot dance until Shiva allows it: He awakes from His ecstasy and, dancing, sends pulsing waves of a sound which awakens the inert matter; even the inferior

matter starts to dance, appearing as a halo around Him. He supports His multiple phenomena through dance. At the peak of time, He destroys all forms and names with fire and concedes further rest. This is poetry, yet this is also science.*

Desacralized therapy has an anti-aesthetic function as regards the voice of Poseidon and the divinities who beckon us to perform the sacred rite and to restore the universal balance. This voice is like a vibration, an inner roaring. This roaring frightens us because we can no longer understand it. We are no longer able to understand the voice of nature, because we expect to have pure mental control over it. We thus become environmentally incompatible creatures, through our own choice of exclusion.

If desacralized therapy is an anaesthetic effort, the sacred ritual is an aesthetic experience of celebration and nobility of the Divine roaring.

The aesthetic experience is the great alternative to therapeutic models. It shifts the emphasis from mental categories of good and evil, health and disease, to pure natural beauty, which is immeasurable, unpredictable, incalculable, just like the fundamental building blocks of matter, the quanta, the tiny agglomerates of energy.

Even though quantum physics is at the base of all of today's science—indeed the properties of quanta not only explain the atomic and subatomic world but also reveal many aspects of astrophysics and cosmology and interpret phenomena in the fields of biophysics, genetics, and neuroscience—it is still little known. This is due to the fact that the ideological implications that it triggers are destabilizing, to say the least, for the medical-sanitary establishment, and consequently for the economies of the nation-states.

Therapy can become ritual when the sick person rediscovers the

---

*Ananda K. Coomaraswamy, *The Dance of Shiva* (Milano: Luni, 1997), 83.

sacred within and offers an unconditioned "Yes" to the call of the soul, giving up oneself to invisibility, to mystery, giving up control over one's own "I." Only then can the sick person turn surgery or a shamanic ritual into a true healing process. Healing is never induced from the outside. The sick person heals because he or she rediscovers the sacred within, thus the therapy becomes a rite of passage whereby the universal order is reestablished.

To heal, not always and not necessarily, means to stay on this side of the Great Threshold and, in any case, to acquire the ability to see that shadow is light; it means to overcome the fear that blocks our awareness of the vanishing of apparitions; it means to acquire the ability to stay vigilant and attentive about the images vanishing and the shadows approaching. The final discovery is that in the vanishing there is self-giving, there is love, which is true life, and ongoing regeneration.

The Mother Mantra Practices Are Rituals, Not Therapies

We can only heal ourselves. As Carriers and Guardians of the Mother Mantra tradition we may pass on healing practices whose function it is to open the channels to the revelation of light, to ideas—gods—so as to make the healing process feasible.

The Carrier of the Mother Mantra tradition is more like a priest who celebrates a rite rather than a therapist. The Carrier is an alchemist who reveals the seven messengers of Hades, transforming the seven demons into the most powerful allies and most faithful protectors. Such a one is able to open up to the sacred in sex, illness, pain, aging, death, sleep, and research, turning these activities into the key to self-giving, to overcoming the cage of the "I" and the walls of individualism; turning them into a means for reestablishing the universal order, the primeval balance, which is ecstasy, immovable pleasure, and freedom.

COMPASSION

Quanta are waves that act like particles when they are observed. Equally, pleasure is like pain when it is perceived, or like a fleeting instant that is lost. This happens because

1. The seven great messengers are misunderstood by our senses. The human senses are corrupted by a subconscious programming, a perceptive filter conditioned by common values. Sight, hearing, touch, taste, and smell are mental operations through which we choose our own manner of interpreting the sensory world out of an infinite number of possibilities. Humans have a penchant for clouding over the senses, for mystifying the truth.
2. The seven great messengers are aspects of the raging Poseidon, who is also Zeus, also Hades, and also Dionysus. The gods are our organs, they are nature, they are matter, they are quanta. There is a willpower in nature.

Nature is soul, spirit, and is pervaded by the gods. The metaphysical God of monotheist religions, who resides in a faraway sky separate from nature, is a human idea—as the renowned priest and theologian Raimundo Panikkar often stated. Placing God in a faraway, metaphysical, transcendent sky was accomplished by the will of humans to gain power and control over nature, the body, and over others. This idea has lent itself to support the set of values of good and evil upon which empires and power are founded.

To bring the Father back into the body of the Mother, to reunite divinity and nature, to accomplish the Mystical Marriage, the alchemical wedding, in our body, in our mind, and in the images that we inhabit—that is, in the world—is a fundamental process for soul-making and for deep ecology, and it is the path for converting pain into pleasure.

Human suffering, generated by the dimming of the senses, produces sorrow, contrariety, disappointment, and bitterness in all of nature, because nature is compassionate. Universal compassion is a fundamental trait of complexity. Given that it is true that the part is in everything and everything is in the part, it is also true that the suffering of one is the suffering of all. Nature suffers because humans suffer; nature dies because humans die.

Yet there is a remedy for this state of suffering and dying, in which death is experienced in unawareness and in pain, as an end, a privation, a halt. We must accomplish the promised rite, which is as yet unaccomplished, and reestablish the universal order, the primeval balance. To do so we must let go of fear and look into the depths of our own suffering, and then go deeper, beyond the barriers imposed by the conditioning of the senses, by discriminating judgment, by analysis. The analysis of perceptions is triggered and dominated by fear. We must overcome it and allow pain to speak for itself and tell its own story. Then we will understand that our pain derives solely from our stubborn will to keep control, to have a deceptive power over nature, over the body, over others. If we let go of this maleficent need, we may then say "Yes" to the call of the soul and accomplish the unaccomplished sacred rite, give ourselves, offer ourselves, vanish and disappear. In the annihilation of the "I" we will rediscover our own Self, the radiant and immortal soul.

We don't know who we really are. Compassion is one of the keys that can open the door to our own self-discovery. Compassion is Sameness. Observing this sick and suffering planet we must realize that we are also observing ourselves. For love's sake we must take on the task of transforming pain and death, for love of the tiger, the golden eagle, the wolf, which are disappearing because, like any aspect of nature, they can only exist on this planet out of love.

For the love of the ant, the dewdrop, the snowflake, a leaf, or a breath of wind, we must become alchemists and transform our own egocentric suffering into a force of love that can accomplish magic.

The Mother Mantra path, like all great spiritual paths, such as full attention and meditation in Buddhism, teaches us to delve deeply into the bodily sensations without judgment. If we investigate a bodily sensation of suffering without judgment we realize that pain and suffering don't actually exist as such. Exploring the painful or fastidious feeling of one's body, the meditator encounters the dance of the elements (earth, wind, fire, water); one meets the feeling of heat and cold, heaviness and levity, dampness and dryness, and so on, but does not meet pain. Pain is an erroneous interpretation of pleasure by the senses that have been corrupted by a subconscious programming, induced by the fear of the organs, which are gods, and by the terror of nature, which is the soul.

The fear of the soul is the reason for the existence of pain. The opportunity to experience the body as a vehicle of pure pleasure, unconditional love, and cosmic union is reason for the existence of the body.

Physical pain stems from the ignorance regarding the four elementals (earth, wind, fire, water), which are perceived as material objects rather than experiences of love. Because love is self-giving, and because self-giving frightens the individual who feels self-attachment, when the body expresses its capacity to self-give, this is perceived as pain, when in truth it is love and pleasure.

Psychological pain too stems from being victims of the materialistic illusion, from the inability to see events as beings, spirits, divine presences, gods, and demons; that is, images devoid of substance and objectivity, creations made up of the same evanescent fabric of dreams. Forgetting to be the dreamer of the dream comes from there, as does the impossibility of interacting with events, which we succumb to as unavoidable objective creations. Frustration, victimization, and annihilation manifest with the unavoidability of events. Forgetting to be the dreamer, we fall victim to our own dreams.

Illness is always the soul's call to the sacred. To succumb to illness means to get trapped while vying for control.

Aging is the symbol of impermanence, which concerns all the manifestations of nature. By refusing to see the impermanence of oneself, trying to stay young whatever the cost, we are condemned to death, because that which remains crystallizes and becomes heavy, material, objective. Objects are inevitably subject to time and die. That which is impermanent appears and vanishes with the speed of lightning, of a quantum of energy, of a wave in emptiness: it appears, vanishes, appears. There is never a death, because there is never actually a true birth, but only an apparition devoid of substance.

Death is a bad cultural habit. Today's individuals have created a culture that is a bullish act of violence on nature. Yet nature is a psychic dimension: we project ourselves in nature and inhabit our own images. The image of death we succumb to is the consequence of our will for power and control, which leads us to experience separateness and fear.

Death stems from the feeling of guilt, from the original sin that the individual harbors for having betrayed the pact with nature. The sin generates fear, and in turn fear generates the impossibility of understanding the shadow, the inability to experience the underworld dimension. It is this incapacity that humans call death.

RITE AND MYTH

The development of archetypal psychology was an extraordinary event in the history of humanity because it showed us the power of mythology. "We can only do in time what the gods do in eternity," wrote the renowned psychoanalyst James Hillman, meaning that the psyche is shaped on original images called archetypes, such as immortal mythical gods, Titans, nymphs, giants, and centaurs. A myth is always rich in drama because it narrates the beauty of nature, which is self-giving, which is sacred.

The mythological drama is painful, as long as an individual succumbs to the intensity of the messengers: the force of suffering, of illness, the unavoidability of death, the impermanence of an orgasm, the effort of research, the darkness and loss of control during sleep. The drama becomes a pure protective and allied energy, an erotic-creative force, only when the individual abandons the role of victim, which in turn is feasible only if accomplished through a rite.

When awareness meets willpower in Shambhala—a state of being, a land beyond space and time, in another high level of energy vibration, the great no-man's-land—a person can "see" the myth that one is enacting on the stage of life. This vision becomes the healing process in itself, according to psychoanalysis. In truth, "seeing" that indeed life is a myth, and understanding which gods, which archetypes, are most active in one's own life still isn't enough to bring about an authentic change. That is not enough to change the course of events, unless one knows how to speak to the gods through the rite. This is the art of magicians and poets. It is the art of love.

Alchemical transmutation requires a ritual. When the myth was separated from the rite we lost our capacity for wanting in unison with the shadow, which has the power to make events happen. The gods are not only to be known, they are also to be loved. It is not enough to perceive them; we must unite with them carnally, with every cell of our body, just as the Canticle of Canticles and the mystics of every esoteric religion of the world invite us to do. This is the tantric rite of the mystical marriage, to which the Mother Mantra tradition is inviting us.

Only the lover of the gods may interpret the myth. Only the Pythia may give voice to Apollo. One of the main problems in today's society is that so many feel authorized to act as Apollo's spokesmen. This is the harmful result of institutions that give out certifications, diplomas, acknowledgments, and permits galore. Only Apollo can choose his own messenger.

Knowledge of the myth cannot be compared to technical knowledge. A multi-specialized graduate, fully qualified for his profession, is not necessarily capable of speaking with the gods, which are organs and ideas. Our civilization has lost the rhythms and harmony of nature and allows false prophets to guide it. Knowledge separated from love is always a double-edged weapon.

The myth in itself is an empty box. The real value is in the voice of the narrator: that voice may fully express Apollo and the force of change, or be learned yet sterile. We need magicians and poets, bards and storytellers who know how to narrate fables of power in a true ritual. These are the same stories that were told in ancient times, in tribes, by expectant mothers so that the newborn might become great. We call these bards Carriers and Guardians of the Mother Mantra tradition. They are the imaginal beings who can bring about a true revolution.

The myth is not a product of reason, so it cannot be investigated with analytical thought. It is *pòiesis,* creation of the soul. The myth contains the original models, which are subject to civilizations, differing cultures, and the life of every individual. The myth has always been entrusted with traveling poets, singers, musicians, and artists. The myth only really comes back to life through oral transmission.

We are in need of bards who know the enchantment of storytelling and who can invent heart-stirring rituals with their magic flutes.

7

Freeing the Hostage Prometheus

THE MYTH OF PROMETHEUS

Prometheus was one of the Titans, son of Iapetus and of the Oceanid Clymene, or Asia. He didn't take part in the battle that arose between the Titans and the Olympian gods, headed by Zeus, because he foresaw his defeat, as established by Fate. Indeed Prometheus, as the name suggests (in Greek, "he who knows before"), is a soothsayer. As a prize for siding with the gods, when the latter vanquished the Titans and plunged them into the Tartarus, condemning them to never-ending punishment, he was allowed free access to Mount Olympus, home of the gods. Thanks to his vicinity to the gods, he witnessed the birth of Athena from the head of Zeus. Athena was very generous with Prometheus and gifted him with wisdom and knowledge of the arts and crafts.

One day Prometheus modeled a man out of clay and brought him to life with the divine flame. Excited about his own beloved creation, Prometheus smothered him with all sorts of gifts and enclosed all the possible evils in a vase, out of man's reach.

At that time men were allowed access to the gods' presence and took part in their gatherings. During one of their feasts, held at Mekone, an ox was sacrificed and its meat was offered to men and gods alike. The head of Olympus entrusted the task of sharing out the meat to Prometheus, who took advantage of the occasion to take revenge on Zeus for having wiped out the Titans in battle.

He slaughtered the animal and sawed it into chunks, keeping back the choicest morsels for the men, hiding the pieces under the disgusting skin of the ox's belly. For the gods he prepared the bones, disguising them in hunks of fat. Once the portions were made he invited Zeus to choose his part and leave the rest for the men. Zeus accepted and chose his part of fat and bones; then, realizing that he had been tricked, he uttered a curse against humankind. Ever since then humans have always left the inedible parts of the animals to the gods, keeping the meat for themselves. But the meat-eaters became mortal because of Zeus's curse. Furthermore, Zeus confiscated fire from men.

Tremendously afflicted by the great suffering of his own creation, and knowing full well that men could not survive without fire, Prometheus decided to steal the fire from the gods and give it back to the men.

Zeus was furious and ordered Hephaestus, the god of metalworking, to forge the statue of a woman, considered the first human female, Pandora. The king of the gods breathed life into the statue and gave her the very vase in which Prometheus had trapped all the evils of humankind, forbidding her to open it. He then summoned Hermes to take her to Earth. During the journey Hermes gave her Curiosity as a gift, before delivering her to Epimetheus. At first Epimetheus refused to welcome her, as he had been warned by his brother Prometheus to accept no gifts from the gods.

In response to this, Zeus ordered Hephaestus to tie Prometheus to a high cliff where an eagle came to feast on his liver every morning. The organ of the Titan regenerated continuously, to be freshly devoured every day.

Epimetheus, saddened by the fate of his brother, gave in and wed

Pandora. Driven by Curiosity, Pandora opened the vase in which Prometheus had enclosed all the evils that might afflict humankind. Epimetheus closed the vase, but it was too late and the evils had already been let loose. Only Hope was left in the vase. The world became a desolate and inhospitable place after the opening of Pandora's vase. According to some versions, Pandora opened the vase a second time, letting out Hope, which was supposed to comfort humanity.

The idea that before the creation of Pandora there were no other women and that humankind was made up of men only is unacceptable, inasmuch as the masculine cannot exist if not in juxtaposition to the feminine and vice versa. In other words, the opposites cannot exist if not contemporaneously.

So, what does it mean to call Pandora the first woman? What does she represent? The creation of the first woman represents, first of all, the birth of the discriminatory consciousness that distinguishes the feminine and the masculine, the Father and the Mother, good and bad, health and disease, and so on. From that moment on the opposites became distinct and separate in the human mind. In truth, the opposites are distinct but not separate and not separable. Indeed, the sufferings of humankind stem from the fact that the human mind discriminates the opposites and forces the senses to perceive a deceptive reality in which the opposites are distinct and separate.

The birth of Pandora represents the initial detachment of humans from the natural state and the entrance of the discriminating mind into an artificial state, where knowledge is generated in an effort of analysis, of control over nature, and of illusory power. In this sense Pandora may be likened to Eve, biting into the fruit from the tree of knowledge.

Pandora symbolizes the earth, which, separated from the spirit, is perceived by the mind as inert matter, devoid of soul, an exploitable resource.

How should we interpret the presence of Hope in the vase?

The issue is certainly linked to the meaning of the word *elpis,* generally translated as "hope," even though it may take on different meanings in Greek ("expectation, solicitude, fear," and also "opinion, thought"), not all necessarily positive; the verb *èlpo* covers an ample semantic area, with various meanings such as "to hope, to expect, to suppose, to think." So, depending on the viewpoint, "hope" may be perceived as a passive and useless illusion or as a supporting force in the face of adversity, encouraging us to move on and better our condition. The fact that elpìs was enclosed in the vase leads to the presumption that it was seen as an evil.

Let's see what the philosopher Nietzsche had to say about hope:

The Greeks differed from us in their appreciation of hope: it was perceived as blind and insidious; Hesiod spoke of hope harshly in a tale and, in truth, he touched on something so unusual that none of today's scholars has understood him. Indeed, this goes against the modern spirit which, with the birth of Christianity, has learned to consider hope as a virtue. Instead the Greeks—who didn't see why they should be left out from future knowledge, on the contrary, they often put questions to the future as a form of religious duty, whereas we are content with hope—so for the Greeks, thanks to all the oracles and soothsayers, the value of hope had to be downgraded, and took on a malevolent and dangerous hue.*

Hope can certainly be seen in two ways: as a passive illusion or as a force of expectancy in faith. Christianity, according to the times, events, and above all its interpreters, can lead one to apply the word *hope* in either way. We don't want to discuss this issue here.

A myth is not a description of reality that may undergo judgment. A myth brings things into being; it is a creative act. In the myth of Prometheus, the gift of divination—an endowment of humans at the

_____

*Friedrich Nietzsche, *Aurora, Thoughts on Moral Prejudices* (Milan: Adelphi, 1964), 34.

time they lived alongside the gods and Prometheus—is taken from the gods, and Prometheus is enchained "somewhere else." With the loss of the gift of divination, hope is all that is left for humans to make what they want of it: a passive illusion or a powerful faith.

Yet the main point is that if the art of divination was once an endowment of humans, then it may be restored.

The story of Zeus's punishment of Prometheus tells of the replacement of the ability to foresee—the enchainment of Prometheus—with hope. Zeus—representing the new power installed after the repression of the underworld chthonian forces (Titans)—substitutes the human capacity of divination with the expectancy that comes with hope.

Since then our great challenge has been to free ourselves of the hypnosis of hope and regain the skill of divination.

"The secret method is to harbor neither hope nor fear," declares the renowned tantric teacher Machig Labdrön.

RESILIENCE IN IMPRISONMENT

Now, imagine a human being with the elegance of a leopard, the strength of a tiger, the dexterity of a gazelle, the wings of an eagle, the invisibility of a chameleon, the power of an elephant, the vastness of a sunset, the silence of a snowflake, and the delicacy of a butterfly. Observe the resilience—that is, the reactivity in the face of adversity—that is inborn in nature. Generally speaking, resilience is the capacity of a system to overcome a change in a positive manner, to self-mend after damage.

The term *resilience* generally refers to metallurgy. Indeed it derives from the study of materials and indicates the property that some materials have of maintaining their own structure or of reacquiring their original form after being crushed or deformed. Thus resilience is a fundamental property in alchemy, in the process whereby common metal is transformed into gold. In a more ample sense, it refers to the art of adapting to change, turning uncertainty into opportunity and risk into innovation.

When applied to humans, resilience indicates the ability to face stressful or traumatic events and the ability to reorganize one's life in a positive manner when met with difficulty; it indicates the strength to react to adverse conditions and overturn them. A resilient person is someone capable of adapting to a given situation, offering a reactive response. The closer a person is to nature the more resilient he or she is. In all of its forms, from the most complex and evolved to the most simple and primitive, nature offers extraordinary forms of resilience.

The capacity for resilience depends a lot on the way challenges are faced. Nature is permanently in a fighting condition. Being in nature necessarily means to be in a fighting mode. Whether you are a leopard or a gazelle, the first thing you must do when you wake is to start running. And the same goes for humans. The difference between us and animals is that we always hope to better our own natural condition, while being fearful of not managing to do so and of succumbing to it. In nature there is no hope; there is rather only the existing moment, to be lived fully, impeccably, without judgment, to be lived with the ability to give oneself up to the eternity of the present instant.

It is possible to develop the capacity of resilience and divination by delving into the subterranean depths of the psyche, which are myth, *poiesis* (creative production), poetry, and soul.

THE FINAL LIBERATION

One fine day Prometheus—who represents our wild soul, our subterranean, instinctive, chthonian part, the Titan who is in the depths of our psyche—will be set free. How? There are different versions of the myth of the liberation of Prometheus. This is obvious, bearing in mind that the myth is our psyche—that is, our soul—and it isn't subject to globalization or standardization.

The myth of Prometheus is one of the most ancient, traced back in many differing forms. The heart of this narrative seems to be the Caucasus, with its complex mosaic of populations: from Georgia, to Azerbaijan, Russia, Abkhazia, Chechenia, to Circassia, and so on. It was precisely on the Caucasian mountain belt that Prometheus was enchained. According to some variants he was chained in a deep cave; according to others on the top of a high mountain. Many differing versions of the myth of the "enchained hero" have been passed down over the centuries.

Prometheus is the archetype of the outsider, the renegade: he lives with the gods yet he is a Titan, the last of the Titans to be free, creative, intelligent, knowledgeable, and, above all, a rebel in the face of authority. Prometheus is an illogical creature: first he made an alliance with Zeus, betraying his own kind, the Titans, then he betrayed Zeus in vengeance. He was capable of love, capable of a passion so strong and far beyond reason that he was ready to steal for the love of his own creation. Prometheus's behavior is the emblem of creative chaos.

Prometheus represents true knowledge, knowledge surfacing from instinct, from the earth, the bones, bent on the search for truth. Zeus represents power and technical knowledge, bent on power and control.

Prometheus gave humans joy, because he had placed them in a condition of true knowledge, which is union, love, and transformation. Zeus gave humans suffering by sending them discriminatory knowledge, which kindles the illusion of knowing and controlling: knowledge separate from love.

It is difficult, if not impossible, to reconstruct a hypothetical "original myth" of the enchained hero. One often comes upon this figure in Caucasian regions, not only in Hellenic Greece but also in shamanic Siberia. Many myths of Caucasian Asia tell of an enchained hero. One example is Amirani; in the ancient Georgian myth he was condemned to enchainment until the end of the world because of his rebellion against the supreme god. To set himself free he brought the world to an end. Or there is Abrysk'yl, the hero of a myth from Abkhazia, who was condemned to eternal enchainment after challenging the supreme god. He also managed to break free, and his liberation coincided with the start of the golden age for the people of Abkhazia.

In Mongolian and Siberian shamanism we meet the topic of kidnapping and imprisonment of the shaman's soul in the underworld or on the peak of a mountain that marks the world's axis. During the soul's imprisonment the shaman's body sickens and is struck by a very high fever or some terrible illness; he stops eating and becomes delirious. Then, when the soul is set free and returns, the shaman heals and discovers that he is endowed with exceptional powers, including divination.

Going back to the Greek Prometheus, in the lost tragedy by Aeschylus, *The Freed Prometheus,* it is narrated that three thousand years after the imprisonment of the hero, another hero, Heracles, would pass by the Caucasus, shoot the eagle who kept tormenting Prometheus with an arrow, and then break the chains to free him. Prometheus had foreseen this a long time before, at the beginning of his imprisonment, and had told the goddess Ios, who had come to bring him solace.

According to a different narration in the Bibliotheca of pseudo-Apollodorus, the centaur Chiron saves Prometheus, offering his own life in exchange for the freedom of the hero. Chiron is the prototype of the shaman-healer and is considered the father of the healing arts and medicine. He is the teacher of Asclepius and Aesculapius, the gods of medicine. Chiron is the son of Philyra (from the Greek "lime-tree," a plant with calming properties), daughter of Oceanus, and of the Titan Cronos, who turned himself into a horse to seduce Philyra. This explains the immortality of Chiron and the fact that he is half horse and half man. Chiron is also the teacher and friend of Heracles.

One day Heracles clashed with the centaurs and slaughtered some of them. The survivors took refuge in the cave of Chiron. To vanquish them, Heracles shot arrows dipped in the poison of the Hydra, the many-headed serpentine water monster in the land of Lerna. By mistake one of the arrows hit Chiron, who, from then on, longed for death, but he was unable to die, being immortal. This is why Chiron decided to offer his own life to Zeus in exchange for the freedom of Prometheus. The father of the gods, who was particularly fond of Chiron, placed him near to himself in the sky, giving rise to the constellation of the Centaur.

By whichever way Prometheus is set free, his liberation brings purification, change, regeneration, and harmony. The end of the world (a world) and the entrance of the Caucasian hero into the Golden Age are powerful symbols of change. The liberation of the Prometheus who is imprisoned in the depths of the psyche brings a true and powerful change. And not only that . . .

To illustrate yet again the nonlinear, illogical, flexible, nonconsequential, nearly mad behavior of Prometheus: after his liberation he became friends with Zeus again and helped him. Indeed he foresaw that if Zeus were to marry Teti they would have a son who would dethrone Zeus. So Zeus made Teti marry a mortal, so as to avoid her bearing a divine son strong enough to overthrow him, and he married Hera instead.

In its final apotheosis, the myth of Prometheus tells us something extraordinary, which could happen to any of us. Because the psyche is myth, "we can only do in time what the gods do in eternity" (James Hillman). So you too, becoming deeply acquainted with yourself, can free the enchained Prometheus—the apparently obscure, though actually luminous, repressed forces that make you unique, different. You may blend the instinctive subconscious endowments, such as divination (Prometheus), with the conscious mind in a harmonious balance. In this way the promethean forces may help the mind redeem itself, free it from its destiny, help it to come away from suffering and self-destruction, and proceed toward a true victory: then you may live your golden age.

The Mother Mantra tradition offers the help that you have

been looking for to get there; it is the experience of the liberation of Prometheus. After this experience you will find that you gradually become the master of your own destiny, because you will develop the faculty to foresee, to "see before." The hope you harbor will be creative faith, not passive expectation. Your path will no longer be a continuous search but rather an incessant discovery. The liberation of the hostage Prometheus is your mission!

To free Prometheus it is necessary to find within yourself the fearless strength of Hercules. You must be able to sacrifice the attachment to pain (Chiron) that has been passed down by many generations; you must be open to real change, which means the dissipation of your subconscious programming. As is told in the myth of Amirani, the illusory world that governs you must end for the dawn of freedom to shine. This implies the upheaval of your set of values. The foundation for real spiritual revolution is when you stop worshipping the deceptive power of the "I" and start supporting true knowledge—which is not sterile erudition but instead the dialogue with your soul.

THE SPIRITUAL REVOLUTION

Humans are so scared of the truth that they often prefer to succumb to death rather than learn to seek the truth. Summing up what has been said up to now, I should stress that in normal conditions the search for truth and the illusory power of the "I" never meet in our society. The seeker for truth isn't interested in the illusory power of the "I," and vice versa. This is expressed in the myth of Prometheus, where Prometheus is he who knows, whereas Zeus is he who yields power.

Evidently there is power in knowledge, but it is the power of freedom. It is also true that there is a certain knowledge in power, but it is of a technical kind, bent on power itself. In normal conditions, unless one has achieved enlightenment and awakening, one who wields power in our society does not have true knowledge, and one who attains true knowledge does not weild the power of the "I." Such a person knows it is an illusory power and is not interested in it. One who knows is solely interested in knowledge.

Those without true knowledge are eco-incompatible creatures, and as much effort as they might make to save life on the planet, they don't know how. They don't know life, or the planet; they don't really know what nature is. Their power is purely illusory. Every step they take toward environmentalism becomes a boomerang sooner or later, because nature slips from the categories of good and bad and only obeys the rhythms of beauty.

To know nature we must undertake the great journey, the adventure into the underworld. If we want to change for the better and if we want to modify our social and cultural models, we have to change the myth that underlies these models. Those who harbor the true knowledge of the myth and those who talk to the gods, those who know the language of fairy tales and of the poiesis, have access to change. Nature guards its own codes in a very secret place, which very few manage to reach. This place is the imaginal, the Sameness.

Since the universe is a complex reality, similar to a hologram, where everything is in the part and the part is in everything, the magnificent worlds of those who are liberated in life live alongside the world doomed to the holocaust, the world of suffering. The worlds are possibilities, all inside one another. Thus our victimized and suffering life lives alongside our free and joyful life. Individuals usually tune in to one or the other alternately, tending to prefer one over the other.

Those who don't feel happy should learn to tune in more to their free and happy life. Those who don't feel happy and aspire to freedom should give much more value to true knowledge than to money or social power. Only like that will they one day meet the three necessary elements for accomplishing a true and full revolution in their lives and world: the teacher, the initiation or teaching, and the community of awakened beings. Then money and abundance will come as a consequence and will appear effortlessly, without the need to ask.

This doesn't mean that a spiritually oriented person should not be interested in money. That would be a big mistake, leaving the power of money in the hands of the forces of ignorance and arrogance. On the contrary, it is important that spiritual people regain the power over money so as to place it in the hands of the Mother. This is feasible on Earth only by way of a revolution in human values.

True knowledge must receive value in order to become valuable and have more economic worth than an object of consumption. Those who know must be put in the position to make decisions. Today the decision makers have no authentic knowledge. This mirrors the condition of our society, which doesn't know what to do with true knowledge. The power of money is different from the accumulation of money. To regain the power of money means to reestablish the natural flux of abundance in which all one's needs are taken care of without effort. Money is hoarded in the wake of subconscious fear.

First of all, people have to rediscover the power of money in their own lives, by letting love win over fear and thus expressing new social values, values that spring from the ability to see the soul of things, and from ceasing to exploit them as such. If humankind could only understand that objects have a soul and that this soul is the true value of the objects, our economy based on the systematic exploitation of nature would cease abruptly.

The inner and outer, personal and global, revolution is feasible for everyone; it is a radical action that changes one's life and one's world. This is what the practices of the Mother Mantra tradition lead to.

The way of the double M is like an underground passage that leads to the fort. Just as an underground secret passage is of great advantage if you want to penetrate, capture, and destroy the fort, the same may be said for the way of the double M: it offers great advantage to those who wish to conquer the fort, which is the illusory world, and destroy it by destroying all the imaginary bricks that make up the mind.

REVOLUTION IN
THE MOTHER MANTRA TRADITION

The Mother Mantra is an experience of awakening and authentic revolution. Those who really understand the extent of this revolution may understand the priceless value of the mantra. The revolution in the Mother Mantra tradition follows precise paths, each with a precise name and indication. They are the Path of the Great Teaching through Taste, Sight, Feeling, Touch, Smell, and Hearing.

❧ Practice of the Great Teaching through Taste, Sight, Feeling, Touch, Smell, and Hearing

This practice is done with the Mystical Marriage Mantra and is used to focus your conscious attention on your sensations.

When you touch something, at the very moment you touch it, repeat the Mystical Marriage Mantra (AYA SAMAS/SAMAYA), feeling that you are in truth touching an aspect of your mystical bridegroom/bride, which is manifesting through what you are touching.

When you see or smell something, when you taste something, when you hear words or music or sounds, repeat the Mystical Marriage Mantra, feeling that you are actually seeing, smelling, tasting, and hearing your bride/bridegroom in her/his infinite manifestations of love. Doing so with the utmost conscious attention, you come into contact with the pleasure produced by the activity of the senses.

This practice is extraordinary and can be done any time you remember, or when you are in the presence of particular objects, odors, sounds, and tastes, so as to savor life with the utmost intensity.

Your perceptive system will soon get used to a major intensity of expression, and you will find that you live more intensely. You will feel more alive because you are more perceptive.

One who perceives the soul perceives the true nectar of the world and feeds on it knowingly.

Used in this manner, the Mystical Marriage Mantra allows you the power to relate sensually to things, bodies, and places because SAMAS/ SAMAYA is the subterranean aspect of your bridegroom/bride, which manifests in objects, bodies, things, in the shadow of things, in their spiritual dimension, and in their primary essence, the anima mundi.

When the bride/bridegroom is perceived in clothes, the great teaching is in the dressing. when the bride/bridegroom is perceived in sounds, the great teaching is in the hearing. When the bride/bridegroom is perceived in food, the great teaching is in the tasting. When the bride/bridegroom is perceived in visions, the great teaching is in the seeing. When the bride/ bridegroom is perceived in smells, the great teaching is in the smelling.

The Path of the Great Teaching through Dressing

When you put an item of clothing on your body, don't treat the clothing as if it were a mere object but instead as a messenger of the soul, a representative of your underworld bride or bridegroom. Then this piece of fabric will protect you, inspire you, guide you, and embrace you lovingly with the vision of your *daimon* all day long. The *daimon* is a spirit of vibrant energy close by your side related to your soul destiny. A garment is an object of knowledge; its power is tied to its origin, its story, and its mission. Your clothes are the first things people see of you. Through the choice of an object of knowledge such as a scarf, a shawl, or a hat, you may pass on a message of true revolution. The beholder potentiates the object of knowledge precisely by beholding it. The objects of knowledge absorb the energy of the onlooker's eyes and protect one from harmful beings.

The color and warmth of garments is never accidental. They are soul and love. They embrace you; they don't dress you. They caress you; they don't just cover you; they are the hands and fingers of the underground bridegroom, of the invisible bride who needs a disguise to show himself/herself to you. The object of knowledge is not chosen by the eyes in front of the mirror but in the half-light by the heart. It expresses the potential of your underground or celestial bridegroom/bride, so the garment is chosen according to the needs of the soul: a hat for getting rid of depressing thoughts, a cloak for making oneself invisible when necessary and for being acute and visionary. The magic is yours for the taking, if only you decide to stop being exploited. Everything is the result of resolutions. Make the firm resolution right now to stop being exploited, and start your relation with the soul of the world.

The Sexual Rite

Pleasure is very important on the Mystical Marriage Mantra path. Pleasure opens the energetic meridians (nadi) and the energetic centers (chakras), offering a state of flowing creativity. The paths of the great teachings are important, because they increase and maintain a high level of pleasure in the body. As we saw earlier, if the body undergoes a collapse in pleasure, the individual is unconsciously brought to act in a harmful way and becomes ever more entangled in the wheel of *samsara*, illusions. The Mother Mantra practitioner must kindle the flames of desire and pleasure (dumo). Thus the sexual rite may be reinvented, dissolving the bodily object in a more ample spiritual reality. This is done by the repetition of the mantra for the nondispersion of the semen. This mantra maintains the body in a state of pleasure and creativity even after intercourse is over and even if the juice, *rasa* (nutritive fluid), both male and female, has been dispersed for a lack of the ability to retain it.

This very precious mantra is ORARO HEKA. HEKA is the magic of the soul that permeates nature. ORARO is a greeting, a beckoning, and a calling. It should be repeated inwardly during intercourse: ORARO while breathing out, and HEKA while breathing in.

While reciting the mantra, allow your body to melt into the body of your partner, and vice versa, becoming one body. Then allow this one body to melt in the light, forcefully rolling your eyeballs upward under closed eyelids, envisioning a bright light. This will help the subtle energies in the semen and rasa to be withheld and to flow back up to meet the Tig Le, the pearl of light in your forehead, which, when it blends with rasa, generates amrita, ambrosia, the nectar of the gods. Then the amrita, dripping into your body, nourishes it with bliss and unfolds it to the revelation.

With the repetition of the mantra ORARO HEKA during intercourse the one body acts as a tool for the reunion of the Father with the Mother and becomes the stage for soul-making and deep ecology. It is then that having a body acquires true meaning.

Thanks to this mantra, in the face of fear, the Carrier of the Mother Mantra can melt harmful and disturbing apparitions. The mantra ORARO HEKA offers the utmost protection. If whispered to tree trunks, rocks, or the tumbling waters of rivers, this mantra offers a deep sense of communion.

Dimensions of Freedom

The enjoyment of beauty and of the things of the world in the knowingness of the mystical marriage has particular, positive effects. The things of the world, which can otherwise imprison and ruin, may produce positive effects through these practices, if done correctly. The passions tied to sex, which generally pull a person into an animalistic state, may raise one to divinity if they are purified and modified through the experience of the mystical marriage.

With these practices not only sensations but also every deep emotion tied to passion, pain, fear, and so on may produce a supreme sense of liberation: the intensity of the emotion may calm mental activity and create an unperturbed state of mind. Even fear, if nurtured and consciously and attentively felt, can become a powerful ally. We are oppressed by fear until it is subconscious and we ignore what we are afraid of. If fear is consciously nurtured it reveals our state as dreamers who forget that they are dreaming, thus becoming victims of the images they themselves have produced.

Considering that things do not have an objective and absolute nature and that those same things in the presence of the mystical marriage, instead of plunging the mind into the world of sorrow, may raise it to supreme bliss and to the final liberation, then even pleasure from touch may produce a similar result. In a state of ignorance this pleasure may condition you or deceive you, but in the awareness of the mystical marriage it may lead to freedom. It all depends on your motivation, mental attitude, and resolution. If the mental attitude is pure, then everything will do yourself and the world good.

Through these practices tactile pleasure can induce a state of marvelous mental balance in which serenity is a natural consequence of the tactile pleasure itself. Just as the arts, through sounds and images, may gradually lead to a serene, solid, and steadfast condition, so may tactile pleasure do the same. This becomes possible only when—with the help of the Mother Mantra teachings—the fundamental nature of things and the world is recognized as void. Then when Mother Mantra practitioners touch, see, smell, taste, and hear, they will understand that their true relation is not to the object itself—which is illusory—but to the soul of the world, which is expressed through the magical apparitions we call objects or individuals.

8

Further Spiritual Practices for Well-Being

MAKING ACQUAINTANCE WITH THE ORACLE

In the real depths we already know which mytheme—the powerful, dramatic, poetic human theme—we are acting out on the stage of life. But to see it and master it is quite something else. To see, we must overcome fear.

From the time of her own adolescence, a mother carries in her heart the countenance of her future children. We carry all the images of our fate in our bowels: the image of the house in which we will live, the family we will have, the way we will die.

There is a soothsayer, a Prometheus, an oracle within each one of us, with a voice like the Delphi Oracle, which told Jocasta that her son Oedipus would eventually kill his father and have intercourse with her.

Jocasta, Oedipus's mother, had married Laius, the king of Thebes. The Oracle of Delphi had foreseen that Laius's son would kill his own father and marry his mother. To avoid the prophecy coming true, Jocasta abandoned her son on a mountain with his feet tied and announced his death. But her son was saved and taken to the court of the king of Corinth, where he was given the name Oedipus. And, when he was grown up, he did kill his own father and have intercourse with his own mother, without knowing who they were until it was too late and the deeds were already done.

What might have happened if Jocasta hadn't been afraid? If she had lovingly brought up and taken care of her son? She would have overcome fate! Oedipus would have always known who his father was and would not have killed him by mistake, not recognizing him. And he would have always known who his mother was and would not have had intercourse with her. Perhaps. Or maybe, if his old, sick father had asked his own son to help him die with dignity, Oedipus would have helped him. And maybe he would have loved his mother without that sense of guilt that then pushed him to blind himself and his mother to hang herself. If Jocasta had allowed love to win over fear, she could have written her own destiny in her own way, changing the ending, thereby changing the destiny of the world.

To transform the drama we have to know how to listen to and accept the voice of the oracle that speaks from the depths of the psyche and not act on the impulse of fear.

To free ourselves of our drama is as difficult as it is easy: we need to overcome fear!

To overcome fear we don't need positive thinking; we need poetic thinking, we need love! We must go beyond positive and negative, overcome the opposites and overcome fear.

By understanding what really frightens us and by becoming acquainted with it our eyes will open onto a deeper vision. Instead of offering ultra-efficient techniques to rid ourselves of the child and silence the oracle, the Mother Mantra tradition leads us into the depths to listen to the oracle and to love the child, both of which are our greatest resources.

It is possible to overcome fear and heal our own destiny; we only have to want to do so. Someone said that "magic is the art of mastering change according to will." The Mother Mantra tradition takes us into the world of magic; we are welcome. We only have to want it!

THE ORACLE
SPEAKS THROUGH IMAGES

The oracle speaks to us through the most outstanding images or impressions (*samskaras*) of our life, such as the faces of our ancestors, the images from recurring or important dreams, meaningful illnesses, accidents, strong emotions, talents and abilities, and enemies.

In the Mother Mantra tradition there is a practice known as the Visionary Mandala, Secret Mandala, or Inner Mandala, whereby it is possible to question the samskaras, the strong impressions in our life, and thus contemplate our dominating myth. The technique is described below.

ꙮ *The Visionary Mandala*

On a big piece of paper, draw as big a circle as you can. At the center of the circle draw a small empty square.

Slip into a gentle trance through deep breathing and continual repetition of the Mystical Marriage Mantra, which you whisper to invisibility.

☙ Breathing and Mantra

In the first phase repeat the Mystical Marriage Mantra for a stretch of three minutes, pronouncing AYA while exhaling and SAMAS or SAMAYA while inhaling. As it is neither natural nor easy to inhale while saying a name, it might take a bit of practice. The result is a deep circular uninterrupted breathing through the mouth. In exhalation, contract the abdomen—that is, pull your belly inward—to give a further push to the outward breath.

Breathe in this way continuously for three minutes. You might feel slightly dizzy or feel pins and needles in your hands and feet. If you do, don't become anxious. It is due to the deep oxygenation and is not harmful; indeed it is purifying and oxygenating your body. Obviously the parameters refer to a healthy person.

After three minutes go on to the second phase, in which you breathe spontaneously for one minute with eyes closed and eyeballs turned upward.

Phases one and two are to be repeated three times.

Drawing the Visionary Mandala

Now recall or visualize a symbol that represents a powerful ancestor; that is, a predecessor whose energy or talent may have been handed down to you. You don't have to have directly known this person, and maybe all you know of him or her is family legend, yet you somehow feel that this person's image influences you and he/she is the right personage for your mandala. As soon as the symbol that represents your ancestor reaches you, draw it on whatever part of the circle inspires you instinctively.

Repeat another three cycles of breathing with the Mystical Marriage Mantra and then "channel" the symbol of a recurring or meaningful dream and draw it on the circle wherever you may choose. You may remember dreams that struck you when you were a child, adolescent, or adult. Choose the dream that struck you most.

Carry on in this way, "channeling" and drawing symbols in any or every color for each of the images in the following list.

Powerful ancestor
Meaningful or important dream
Main emotion of your childhood (ask yourself what kind of child you were: Were you mostly sad, rebellious, angry, distracted, lonely . . . ?)
Main emotion of your adolescence
Main emotion of adulthood (if you have already lived long enough to be able to define it)
The greatest lack you have felt from childhood up to now
Your animal spirit (which animal, where does it live, what is it like?)

Your biggest loss

The talent you would like to activate

The emotion that would surface if you were to tell of your birth

Your most meaningful illness or accident

All of these impressions (samskaras) are messengers from the king or queen of the shadows—Samas or Samaya—and they speak to you about the myth that you are enacting on the stage of your life. They are depicted in symbolic and instinctive forms in the Visionary Mandala.

How does a myth speak? Certainly not in a manner that common thought might understand. When you contemplate the symbols on the mandala, you have to give up understanding them. They are not concepts, they have no meaning; rather they are forces that need to be liberated.

᚛ The Contemplation of the Visionary Mandala

Now hang the drawing on a wall so it will be straight in front of you about three feet away when you sit in a position for meditating.

Observe it through half-closed eyes, without adjusting the focus, breathing in a circular fashion as described in the first phase of the practice, "Breathing and Mantra."

Stay in this contemplation for ten to twenty minutes.

You may repeat this contemplation after a month or two. Each time you do this practice you can focus on a different symbol of your mandala, evoking its memory, power, voice.

Every person, event, or place symbolized on your Visionary Mandala is thus subtracted from the domain of objectivity and materialism. Now that it is on your mandala it is openly a symbol, an image, a dream. And when you sit contemplating the mandala, you are the dreamer who is aware of the dream, and you have power over the images. This is the reabsorption of reality. The liberation of the deep psychic contents and energies happens in increasing intensity and is renewed every time. In the beginning reality is reabsorbed in an "imaginal creation." Further on, the necessary energies to act on the imaginal creation are awakened.

THE IMPORTANCE OF FOOD HABITS

You may remember the promises that keep alive the memory of the spirit of the Mother Mantra, which were mentioned in chapter 5 as the "Practice of Remembrance."

The sixth promise was as follows: "AYA SAMAS/SAMAYA, I promise to follow a healthy diet, AYA SAMAS/SAMAYA."

A healthy diet is not only good for your body's health but also because it expands the heart's capacity and helps the mind gather inspiration with clarity and acumen. An inspired life is the result of a combination of many factors, and a healthy diet is undoubtedly one of the most important. Ideas are eidola, gods. To gain the favor of the gods a healthy diet is a must, putting the body in a non-inflammatory, peaceful, and serene condition in harmony with the rest of nature.

Red meat is without a doubt one of the most inflammatory foods and should be avoided. Dairy products, which also inflame and irritate the organs, should be cut down. Eggs aren't easily digested and cause toxin accumulation.

A Mother Mantra Carrier should definitely avoid refined flour. Bread, pasta, and cereals should always be whole-grain and organic. A refined grain brings with it a feeling of separation, division, and dismay because it has been separated from its own husk.

The Mother Mantra Carrier's diet is rich in fruits, vegetables, and legumes.

Following are the basic guidelines for a healthy diet.

- Avoid meat, dairy products, and eggs.
- Avoid refined sugar.
- Avoid coffee, fizzy drinks, and alcohol.
- Strongly reduce the consumption of nightshade plants because they contain solanine, a toxic alkaloid that weakens the immune system. Some of the most common nightshades are the potato, bell pepper, chili pepper, tomato, and eggplant.
- Drastically reduce fried food.
- Consume the season's fruits and vegetables, whole-grain cereals, legumes, and seeds.
- Fish may be eaten once or twice a week at the most and should never be fried, grilled, or smoked. The best way to cook fish is by steaming or under salt.
- Avoid butter, lard, margarine, tinned sauces, refined salt.
- For sweetening, as an alternative to refined sugar, use barley malt or rice malt.
- Suggested seasonings: raw salt, soy sauce, tamari, miso, top-quality vegetable oils, and sesame seeds.

There is no reason for healthy food to not be tasty and enticing. Good food can be both healthy and delicious. It's definitely worth taking time to learn how to cook healthily, to go to the market and personally choose healthy and nutritious foods that you would like to prepare for yourself and your loved ones.

THE WILD SOUL AND THE LOVE FOR YOUR OWN BODY

Unless you are able to recognize and love diversity, the wild soul—which always represents diversity—will always be put to a disadvantage by the educational process.

The ability to recognize your own wild soul and to back your own diversity is in part inborn and in part upheld by the family. This is rare. Generally speaking, especially during the age of development, your own peculiar traits are seen as fastidious characteristics that might even hinder a successful life later on. Deceptively it would seem that conforming to the given model of success might increase your chances of success, whereas this is not at all true. Unconsciously you are led to sedate, if not punish, the wild soul when it rears up and shows its impatience for a "limited" life, when it shows its "difficult" and "weird" ideas, when it shows its diversity.

In an interview with Pier Paolo Pasolini, the Italian poet Giuseppe Ungaretti said that civilization is an act of tyranny against nature. Unknowingly, individuals favor this act of violence toward their own wild soul.

Sometimes people eat, drink, and smoke to keep this outsider away, this crazy horse that paws, quivers, trembles and fidgets, aching for something more. It is a thousand times better to let the wild soul fidget and break something rather than guzzle alcohol or sugar. To give vent to your wild soul, go for a walk in the woods, run along mountain paths, go skiing or swimming. Don't douse it with toxins by eating badly.

Don't punish the soul by eating poison! Everything industrialized, excessively processed, is poison for the soul because it uproots the soul from its natural context in which it breathes and pulsates.

The stronger your soul becomes the easier it will be for you to eat better, and the better you eat the stronger your soul will become. Then this world, which definitely prefers you to be governable, measurable, and predictable, will have to take stock of your diversity through which you express your mercy and your love.

Above all, hearken to your diversity and make it your greatest patrimony, fearlessly. In the end it's always the outsiders who contribute best to this world, when they manage to emerge, loving themselves and their own wild soul.

HEALING AND DEEP ECOLOGY

At this point of the book you have already received many precious treasures. You have two powerful mantras, the first being the Egyptian Mantra and the second being the Mystical Marriage Mantra. You have the very precious mantra for the nondispersion of rasa, ORARO HEKA. And furthermore you know the marvelous morning and evening spiritual rituals.

Other highly beautiful and effective practices can be learned directly from a Mother Mantra Guardian, who can teach them to you after having passed on to you the Mother Mantra proper, which for now is still traditionally tied to a strictly direct, oral transmission. The Guardian may also teach you the spiritual healing practices that are exceptional systems for healing the body, emotional upsets, the mind, and one's life.

But now I would like to give you a self-healing ritual, which you can perform on yourself or on anyone who needs your help by means of the Mystical Marriage Mantra. This practice works on akasha, the fifth element, ether or space. It not only heals the individual, but, every time it is performed, it heals, harmonizes, and spiritualizes the whole planet. This is why I wish to reveal it in written form, even though it is traditionally passed on orally. I feel I have the consent of the masters, as it is now time for union. There can be no individual healing if the planet is not healed at the same time. The feeling of being finite and shut in oneself is deceptive and a cause for suffering. Now is the time for deep ecology.

Deep ecology is an ecology that keeps its distance from institutionalized anthropocentrically stressed environmentalism and ecologist movements. Deep ecology is expressed through a heartfelt interest for the fundamental philosophical questions about the role of human life as part of the ecosphere, differing from ecology, which is a branch of biological science, and differing from utilitarian environmentalism, which is centered merely on human well-being. Deep ecology makes the effort to go beyond the rationalist duality of the human organism on one hand and its natural environment on the other, allowing attention to focus on the intrinsic value of other species, systems, and natural processes. Deep ecology can offer a philosophical standpoint for environmental legislation, which, in turn, can guide human activity away from self-destruction. Deep ecology is scientifically based on ecology, and systems dynamics on the one hand and, on the other hand, on peoples' ancient spiritual knowledge.

The self-healing practice that I am about to reveal to you is in every sense definable as a practice of deep ecology, because it is performed with full awareness of the indivisible unity of persons and planet.

☌ Ritual of Self-Healing and Deep Ecology

⌒ Preparatory Practice

Sit in a meditation posture.

Place your hands over your belly button. Breathe deeply through the nose synchronizing the silent repetition of the Mystical Marriage Mantra with your breathing: AYA exhaling; SAMAS or SAMAYA inhaling.

Feel the belly move under your hands. When you inhale it swells slightly to make room for the incoming air; when you exhale it empties and contracts slightly to help expel the air. Breathe with your belly and lower lungs; don't involve the thorax or clavicular region.

Feel that your belly is the cave, the cavern, which represents all the caves and caverns on the planet, above sea level and below sea level, full of water underground or in the seas. The cave represents the elements of earth and water. With the mantra send love vibrations to the planet's caves, to the earth and the water.

After a minute, shift your hands to the rib cage and start breathing with the chest. Feel the thorax expand slightly under your hands when you inhale and contract slightly when you exhale. Don't involve the belly or shoulders in the breathing now.

Feel that the movement of your chest is a flame that expands and contracts in the wind. The thoracic space belongs to fire and air. With the mantra send love vibrations to the terrestrial magma, to fire, and to the air, wherever they may be.

After another minute shift your hands to your shoulders: right hand on left shoulder, left hand on right shoulder. Now breathe with the upper part of your body, the clavicular region. Feel the shoulders gently rise when inhaling and gently fall when exhaling. The clavicular cavity represents infinite space, the ether, akasha. With the mantra send love vibrations to the universe.

After another minute lay your hands on your lap, palms up, right hand resting on left hand. Join the three respirations in one big, deep continuous breathing cycle.

Start filling your lungs with the belly, then the thorax, and lastly the clavicular region, without interruption, and then empty your lungs inversely, from the top to the bottom, repeating the Mystical Marriage Mantra all the time and sending love vibrations to your underworld or celestial bridegroom or bride, who is the king or queen of invisibility, the soul of the world. This last phase lasts a minute too.

The whole preparatory phase takes four minutes.

ᔓ Self-Healing through the Marman

The *marman* are areas of the body known in shamanic yoga as "energetic joints," inasmuch as they are points where the main nadi, energetic meridians, meet.

The practice consists of transmitting the vibrations of the Mystical Marriage Mantra to these marman points by tapping them with the tips of the index and middle fingers. Every group of marman tapping is preceded by the repetition of a psychic formula of the imaginal creation.

ᔓ Marman Tapping: Group 1

Recite the psychic formula inwardly, then tap every marman for about thirty seconds, whispering the Mystical Marriage Mantra while you breathe gently and deeply through your mouth.

First psychic formula: *Evoke pleasant memories from your childhood and adolescence. Your mind is about to be deprogrammed; it is important for you now to evoke memories so as to widen the borders of your awareness and allow the energy of the Mystical Marriage Mantra to act throughout the space of your mind.*

First group of marman: nape of the neck, neck, shoulders, coccyx, soles of feet.

Let the vibrations of the Mystical Marriage Mantra penetrate the marman.

❧ Marman Tapping: Group 2

Just as before, repeat the psychic formula inwardly and then, starting with the palms of your hands, tap each marman for about thirty seconds each, allowing the vibrations of the Mystical Marriage Mantra to penetrate, and then move on to the other marman.

Second psychic formula: *Remember that you are loved.*

Second group of marman: palms, ankles, around the knees, elbows, wrists.

❧ Marman Tapping: Groups 3–5

The same scheme is applied for the other formulas and groups of marman, as follows:

Third psychic formula: *Let go now of all the traumatic memories, beliefs, and emotions that hinder your full healing.*

Third group of marman: belly button, heart chakra (center of the thorax), throat, closed eyes.

Fourth psychic formula: *Relax your eyes and enter deeply into peace.*

Fourth group of marman: temples, forehead in the point between the eyebrows, the fontanel on top of the head.

Fifth psychic formula: *Your psyche has been deprogrammed. You are free to be healthy and fulfilled.*

Take some rest, repeating the Mystical Marriage Mantra inwardly.

This simple and effective healing practice may also be offered to others, asking the receiver to lie down. During the preparatory practice the person is asked to lie on his/her back and place their hands on the various body cavities. Then the person places his/her hands straight alongside the body. The Mystical Marriage Mantra Carrier then takes over and taps the points of the person's body corresponding to the marman. For the time it takes to go over the first two groups of marman the person lies face downward, whereas for the rest of the groups the person lies on his/her back again.

Healing, or self-healing through self-tapping, may be performed at any time of the day. In the morning it has an energizing effect; done in the evening it has a relaxing effect. Regular practice greatly improves the quality of life. Hopefully this practice will spread and catch on quickly for the benefit of the planet and everyone on it. It could trigger a real spiritual revolution if enough people (the critical mass) are reached. Let's hope it happens soon, for the sake of peace and freedom.

THE ORACLES

In the Mother Mantra tradition, the so-called oracles are extraordinary meditations that the Guardians know, practice, and teach.

I would like to end this book about the Mother Mantra with a description of one of the oracles I love most. The practice of this meditation could be defined, in pure shamanic style, as a ritual for hunting the soul. In deep psychology it would be described as a reintegration practice. It doesn't matter which terminology you prefer to use, because the Mother Mantra is a universal tradition and in the end what really matters and makes the difference is that it is actually practiced. The difference between someone who repeats the mantra several times during their day and someone who does not is immediately evident. You can tell by their eyes, their skin, their smell. Michael often told me that the

Mother Mantra Carriers emitted an incenselike fragrance. For many years I believed his words were symbolic; now I know that he meant it literally.

⋎ The Oracle of Love

Sit in a posture for meditation and whisper the Mystical Marriage Mantra to the invisible for a couple of minutes while asking your underworld bride/bridegroom to lead you into the underworld, the universe of invisibility, the reign of the soul. The Mystical Marriage Mantra practiced with deep breaths induces a gentle trance, an amplified state of consciousness, which allows the ritual to be most effective.

↶ Love for the Newborn You

Come into contact with a fragment of your soul that resides in the world of invisibility. This fragment is yourself as a newborn baby. If you breathe deeply you can see yourself as a newborn baby and in the very first days of your life. You may also see yourself in the fish state in the intrauterine phase of your life. This is a fragment of your soul that resides beyond the Great Threshold, in the realm of Hades. You can take possession of this fragment if you manage to give up the battle that this world is fighting out of fear against the soul.

Produce and contemplate an image of yourself in the intrauterine phase and in the first days of your life. Try to feel what the main emotions and sensations of this creature were, its mission and what your guiding spirit whispered then in your ears.

Reabsorb this image of your embryonic and newborn self with the following psychic formula of the imaginal creation.

Exhaling pronounce the formula: *I love you unconditionally.*
Inhaling, pronounce *your name* (keep up the exercise for a couple of minutes).

ᕙ Love for the Child You

Now take up the Mystical Marriage Mantra, still breathing deeply through your mouth. For two minutes create and contemplate the image of yourself as a child.

Call the child you were back from the reign of shadows; remember your face, your feelings, your games, your favorite places, favorite tastes; and reabsorb it all through the psychic formula of the imaginal creation.

> Exhaling, pronounce the formula: *I love you unconditionally.*
> Inhaling, pronounce *your name* (keep up the exercise for a couple of minutes).

ᕙ Love for the Adolescent You

Now take up the repetition of the Mystical Marriage Mantra again, breathing through your mouth. Visualize yourself as an adolescent. Evoke this fragment of your soul, the adolescent you were. With the help of the Mystical Marriage Mantra and the deep breathing you will gradually see yourself as an adolescent. Observe the feelings you had, the places you knew, the friends you had. The repetition of the Mystical Marriage Mantra leads you deeply into the emotions.

Reabsorb the adolescent you were with the help of the psychic formula of the imaginal creation.

> Exhaling, pronounce the formula: *I love you unconditionally.*
> Inhaling, pronounce *your name* (keep up the exercise for a couple of minutes).

ᕙ Love for the Adult You

Now take up the repetition of the Mystical Marriage Mantra again, breathing through your mouth. Concentrate on another fragment of your soul: the adult, the grown-up, mature person. Observe the thoughts, the emotions, the trials, the joys, and anything else you can evoke. Thanks to the repetition of the Mystical Marriage Mantra this fragment leaves the realm of invisibility, and you may reintegrate it.

Reabsorb it with the help of the psychic formula of the imaginal creation.

Exhaling, pronounce the formula: *I love you unconditionally.*
Inhaling, pronounce *your name* (keep up the exercise for a couple of
minutes).

ᐁ Love for the Elder You

Now take up the repetition of the Mystical Marriage Mantra again, breathing
through your mouth. Evoke yourself in old age; you can feel the emotions and
moods, and once again the guiding spirit whispering in your ear. Take the images from the realm of invisibility, make them visible, may the invisible be seen!

Reabsorb the image of yourself in old age with the help of the psychic
formula for the imaginal creation.

Exhaling, pronounce the formula: *I love you unconditionally.*
Inhaling, pronounce *your name* (keep up the exercise for a couple of
minutes).

ᐁ Full Reabsorption

Now take up the repetition of the Mystical Marriage Mantra again, breathing through your mouth. Realize that the name you are reabsorbing, SAMAS
or SAMAYA, is that which you are and that which all of nature is.

Breathe even more intensely while repeating the Mystical Marriage
Mantra, and reabsorb nature itself through the name SAMAS or SAMAYA.
Every tree, the rain, the mountains: every aspect of nature that you can
evoke is now an aspect of yourself; reabsorb the fragments of your soul.

Repeat this formula: *I love you unconditionally* when exhaling, and
Mother when inhaling. Feel the strength, the energy, and the joy that this
reabsorption brings about in you. Carry on for a couple of minutes.

To finish, stay still and breathe spontaneously with your eyes closed until
you deem right for yourself.